Praise for "Caring for the Caregiver"

I learned that I am my most important resource.
Cynthia Reget, MSW, Social Worker, New York City.

This book will help us learn how to think more about our own needs.
Sharon Tsukahara, LPN, Staff Nurse, Honolulu.

I especially enjoyed your straightforward advice on assertiveness, confrontation and self-accountability. If we caregiving professionals were to systematically put into practice all of the guidelines you've laid out for us, we would find that....our lives would change dramatically for the better. And the world around us would change remarkably also.
Patricia Allison, author of ***Hooked But Not Helpless: Ending Your Love/ Hate Relationship with Nicotine.***

This book makes me feel better about myself.
Marvilynne Helm, RN, Traveling Nurse, San Diego.

I would highly recommend this book to anyone who is looking to open their life to the miracles of self-love.
Lori Whittaker, B.S., Addictions Counselor, Portland.

As a comprehensive, easily readable and solution-packed approach to the overwhelming problem of co-dependency in the caregiving professions, I heartily recommend Ms. Jarrett's book.
Rev. Sally Rutis, RN, Associate Minister, Living Enrichment Center, Beaverton, Oregon

Caring for the Caregiver

A Nurse's Journey to Health and Inner Peace

Roberta M. Jarrett

Illustrations by
Katherine Gray

Happy Talk Books
Beaverton, Oregon

ISBN: 0-9635191-0-7
Library of Congress Catalog Card Number: 92-75402

First Printing, January 1993
Typeset by Letter Perfect, Beaverton, Oregon

Published & distributed in the United States by:
Happy Talk Books
2951 SW Cedar Hills Blvd.
Suite No. 161
Beaverton OR 97005

Publisher's Cataloging-in-Publication Data
Jarrett, Roberta M.
Caring for the caregiver: a nurse's journey to health and inner peace/Roberta M. Jarrett.
p. cm. Includes: index; ill.
ISBN: 0-9635191-0-7 : $12.95
1. Nursing - Psychological Aspects. 2. Co-dependency (Psychology). 3. Mind and Body. 4. Women - Spiritual Life. 5. Health.
I. Jarrett, Roberta, 1938- II. Title
610.73 .J1 RT 86 .J1 92-75402

Dedication

It is with much love and appreciation that I dedicate this book to caregivers everywhere. It is my hope and prayer that it will bless you on your journey.

Acknowledgements

I wish to thank the people who have inspired me to reach for my dreams and to persevere in achieving my goals. First and foremost, my husband Bryan for his patience, persistence and dedication to helping me in my work and in my life.

To my beloved family I offer deep appreciation. Special gratitude goes to my daughter Katherine whose companionship has brought me strength and whose wonderful illustrations have captured the essence of my writing. Many thanks to my sons Joseph, Michael and John for their love and encouragement all along the way. I acknowledge my dear sisters Judith and Kate for the very special parts they have played in my growth. My mother has left this life, but I know she is pleased with the way things have turned out for me. I thank both her and my dad for bringing me into this marvelous world and for the lessons they provided. Many thanks also to my step-dad Walter who has always been there for me and to my step-mom Eva who is loving and caring.

To my dear friends who are more like family to me I offer my gratitude. To say thanks to all would require a chapter itself, but special recognition nonetheless is due Margaret Setliffe, Char LaCroix, Elizabeth Mason, and Kathy Yochum.

Thanks as well to the many, many dedicated caregivers in all professions with whom I have been privileged to work over the past thirty years in nursing. I have been blessed by your sharing your experiences, your dreams and your recoveries.

To the many friends and colleagues who read the manuscript and offered valuable criticism and comments I extend my appreciation. A special thanks is due to Dave High for typesetting the manuscript; to Malaura Riley and Mickey Lee for their creative contributions; and to the staff of Gilliland Printing, Inc., for their patience and fine work.

No acknowledgment would be complete without noting the efforts of the friendly and helpful librarians at Beaverton Public Library and Multnomah County Library, Portland. They could always find an answer no matter how obscure or seemingly difficult the request.

Many thanks to my spiritual teachers. Your names are in my book. *Mahalo nui loa* to Renee La Mer for her special assistance. Last but not least I acknowledge the inspiration and counsel given to me by Berdell Moffett and Casey Chaney who showed that it could be done.

Foreword

In the business of taking care of others, we are often not so good at taking care of ourselves. This is the gentle and timely message of Roberta Jarrett's new book. Her message applies to those of us in the spiritual healing business as well as those in the purely physical caregiving areas. The basic theme is thus: before we take care of those we teach or otherwise tend to, we first must learn to take care of ourselves. Her message is certainly a contemporary variant on the ancient adage, Physician, Heal Thyself.

Roberta's volume analyzes this phenomenon unflinchingly. She presents a program for caregivers to learn to how to love and nurture themselves, thus changing the old messages, self-talk and avenues of behavior. It has often been said that insanity is the practice of doing things the same way and expecting different results. If this is indeed the case, then Roberta's book is a model of sanity in its presenting a workable context for doing things and approaching life in *different* ways. We ALL benefit from the inevitable different results.

Every so often a book comes along which professionals in the field say, "I wish I'd had this book when I was starting out," or "this should be required reading for all ...." Roberta Jarrett's masterly and timely *Caring for the Caregiver* is indeed such a text. It is to be savored by health care professionals and laypersons alike, indeed, by all on the journey to wholeness and happiness.

Roberta is obviously a woman of immense resources and draws from a vast reservoir of technical and spiritual knowledge. Yet she wears her wisdom lightly and presents her common sense message with disarming simplicity and readability. Each chapter stands alone as a virtual self-contained clinic itself. The reading lists and workbook sections are especially useful tools.

I am pleased to endorse and introduce this important work and recommend it to all readers. This book might well be described as universally suggested reading as we learn to take better care of ourselves and each other on this planet.

– Alan Cohen
Maui, Hawaii

Table of Contents

Preface

I completed the manuscript for this book when I was working as a staff nurse at the Hansen's Disease Settlement in Kalaupapa, Hawaii. Since that time I have added to my experiences in nursing and revised the manuscript several times. Now it is ready to be born. From the time the writing first began several years ago up to the present, my life has continually changed and improved.

It remains obvious to me, however, that although many caregivers are learning to take better care of themselves, the vast majority are still better at taking care of other people. I believe that there is a need for a commitment to personal health and well being in the BODY, MIND and SPIRIT for every one of us, especially those of us who choose to become professional caregivers.

Since my helping experience has been mainly as a registered staff nurse, my perspective has been from one who has served in that capacity. However, I hope that the messages contained in this book are equally valid for all professions, as well as for volunteers who give so much of themselves in churches and service organizations of all kinds. I have tried to keep my book concise and to the point, as this is but one approach to the infinite subject of the spirit's journey. There are many other books available for those who wish to pursue the topics I have only briefly touched upon. Selected titles are provided in the reading lists at the end of each chapter.

My colleagues have often encouraged me to share more of my experiences and ideas. They were the inspiration for this book. Although there are numerous autobiographical episodes and anecdotes referred to in the text, this book is not a biography in the usual sense. A specific part of my story is covered, in a somewhat more conventional autobiographical format, in the soon to be published book, **Kalaupapa Diary**. Likewise, those readers expecting a prescription to reform the current medical establishment will be disappointed. In the present work the focus is on the individual, what one person can do *in her own life* to improve the situation. Thus, in a very real sense, the messages and comments herein are directed as much to myself as to the reader.

No discrimination is intended by referring to caregivers and health professionals in the feminine. The fact is that most members of the helping professions are women. Further, this practice simplifies the narrative flow. Likewise, the term "God" is referred to in the masculine simply for reasons of simplicity and is not meant to imply any gender favoritism. As much as possible I've attempted to avoid medical terminology and other jargon. In those instances where I've felt an explanation was needed, a footnote or other reference has been provided.

My own transformation began in the area of physical wellness and moved steadily to the emotional and spiritual realms. I structured the book to begin with the physical area, but you may begin in any section. I suggest that you read quickly through the book once. Then go to the chapter which resonates with where you are in your life now. For example, if you are struggling with how to deal with work overload and a demanding employer, you may wish to start with the section dealing with self-care and emotional wellness. On the other hand, if you have decided you may have a problem with chemical dependency, you may wish to focus on that area of the book.

When you focus, I suggest that you read the chapter and then, as honestly as possible answer the questions at the end. Then do the exercises which are suggested. If you want to pursue the topic of a particular chapter further, read some of the books listed as references. I hope they will be a powerful tool to help you direct more of you energies to caring for yourself in healthy, nurturing ways.

It is not always possible for us to change our personal work environment in any major way. It is *always possible* for us to change the way we view that environment. As Johanna Field has described it so well, "There are two entirely opposite attitudes possible in facing the problems of one's life. One to try to change the external world, the other, to try to change oneself."

Roberta M. Jarrett, C.Ht., BSN, RN
Beaverton, Oregon
November 1992

Chapter 1: Sharing My Story

Only by going through our struggles and by sharing them with others so that they can see our victory over them by the power of God in our lives do we become a light for others to follow.

– Ruth Fishel

There is only one success, to be able to spend your own life in your own way.

– Christopher Morley

And the caterpillar said: "But change is such a fearful thing!"

Have you ever felt a sense of futility and emptiness about your life? Have other people often perceived you as being far more capable, successful and attractive than you believe you are? Have you been the kind of person who finds it much easier to take care of other people's problems than your own?

Did you ever think that your life would be happy IF ONLY.....your husband made more money; your home was the biggest and the best one on the block; your children were all at the top of their classes in school; you never made any mistakes; you went more places; you got more attention from other people in the community? Did you ever feel that you were just not working hard enough? Have you sometimes thought you were a failure because you could not anticipate every single problem which might come along so that you could be prepared for it? Have you felt you could not relax completely unless you had just a few glasses of wine or a couple of drags on a cigarette? Did you ever feel misunderstood and unappreciated in your work? Have you ever felt so totally worthless and desperate that you wanted to end this thing called life? I have. I suspect that my story is not unique; that it is shared in some aspects by a great many in the "helping" professions.

I am a caregiver. Not only have I been a professional caregiver, I have been a caregiver in every other part of my life from girl scouts to church worker. I have had great difficulty saying "No" to the needs of others. Even if I became angry and resentful toward those needs, I would do whatever I thought I SHOULD do, rather than what I felt called to do or wanted to do. I was trapped by the idea that I had no value in life unless I could prove I was worthy by my job performance, my achievements, my possessions, my social standing or my service to others.

I did not understand that we design our own experience; that our reality is changeable. Today, I realize that I must be my own best friend in order to be an effective and healthy participant in any role which I take in life. I understand that I have choices. I am responsible for my own happiness. I choose where I want to work and live and I deserve to be happy. I have a job that I love, working with people whom I appreciate, and who appreciate me. Whether I am happy is totally up to me. I no longer need to be angry, resentful, depressed or trapped in unpleasant situations.

It is not possible to love others without judgment until we love ourselves without judgment and with real compassion. It has been a long, arduous journey, the road to self-love. Perhaps by sharing only part of my story and what I have learned, others will be enriched.

One of the first things I did to love myself better was to take up running. At the time I did not realize that just by doing it, I was really *committing* to my well-being. How my life changed when I learned to exercise! I really don't know where I got the idea but when I did things took a major turn for the better. Where the idea came from is not important.

What is important is that I was *ready for change.* Even though the benefits of aerobic exercise had been documented for years I had never quite gotten the message. I was unable to commit to a regular exercise program until I almost died.

I was living in a small Midwestern farming community, married to a successful professional man and the mother of four wonderful children. For five years I had been a full-time homemaker and community volunteer. I thought I was retired from nursing. I was wrong. Two dynamic young doctors moved into the community and our small hospital became a booming business. Instead of going off to other, larger cities for surgery or other treatment, local people opted to remain at home. They came to appreciate the excellent medical care which was being provided. This placed tremendous strain on the hospital staff, especially the nurses. We needed more RN's and I was soon enlisted to return to my profession. I was not at all happy about it. I remember crying as I bought some new uniforms and shoes. But I believed that if I, as a member of the community, expected the hospital to be there and to function for me and my family, I would have to do my part to see that was possible. I agreed to do a couple of shifts a week.

But something amazing happened. After two shifts, I was approached by the administrator and asked to become the first secular director of nurses the hospital had ever had. There weren't enough nuns available anymore. What an ego trip that was! Even though I had a large home, garden, four children, big yard and pool to take care of, I agreed to take on a full time job. I did clear out a lot of extra activities from my calendar, but I still placed very high demands on myself as a parent and homemaker.

Life at the hospital was very busy; it was small, but it provided coronary care, emergency, pediatric, medical-surgical and full obstetrical care. Much needed to be done in order to meet the ever increasing demands being placed on it.

We had to develop a stable and fair staffing system, recruit more professionals, develop a patient acuity system, establish new patient services as well as provide for the daily care of all sorts of patients. Often I had to fill in as staff nurse because there was simply no one else to do it. I did a lot of wonderful things for that hospital; I sacrificed much. I got pretty angry and resentful because I did not know how to say NO. I was a person who took on every criticism and complaint leveled toward anyone associated with me or working under my direction as though it was a personal attack on my own worthiness.

After a year of no respite I went into a tailspin and suffered a classic case of nurse burnout. Interestingly, it was only when the pressure was removed - when I quit my job - that the severe depression really took hold of me. I had a sense of failure and self loathing because I had not measured up to some self-imposed standard of perfection. I could never imagine that just by right of my humanity I possessed inherent value.

In my personal life I still had all that anyone might want - beautiful family, gorgeous home, possessions of all kinds, wonderful travel experiences, money for everything I needed. and I was not happy. My marriage was gradually unraveling, but I was unwilling to deal with that reality for five more years. I had to heal myself and get a lot stronger. I thought that my state was simply the result of what I had gone through at work. The odd thing was that I did not know that I was getting sick. Looking back now, the symptoms are so obvious: inability to sleep; the sense of unworthiness when I entered a room full of people; the constant feeling of sadness; the crying, the extra weight, the lethargy. Nothing had tipped me off that I was suffering from depression. It went on for several weeks while I carried out my daily activities and served as a very active (and very unhappy) church volunteer.

Then one day I woke up. My family had gone off to work

and I knew exactly how I was going to kill myself. I began to cry and knew that I was in deep, dark trouble. Thank God I had enough sense to realize that no one thinks that way who is not very, very sick. I called my doctor and asked for help. He made all the necessary arrangements for me to be admitted to the hospital under the care of a fine psychiatrist. He told me to pack a bag; I would be staying for a few days. That afternoon, my husband drove me to the hospital which was two hours away from where we lived. I thought I would be there for the weekend but I remained for a whole month. I was on suicide precautions for two weeks and I took antidepressant medication for a year.

That episode was pivotal for me. I had to create a shocking experience in order to begin my personal growth. From that day on I learned, gradually, to take care of myself. My life prior to that time had been about trying to please someone else, of meeting some illusive standards of performance which I thought would make me happy. But this is not so. I found that happiness does not come that way. The unique creation, the one of a kind masterpiece which is me (or you), cannot really blossom without our own approval and love. The acceptance of others may come but it cannot be the primary source of our happiness.

It was after I came home from the hospital that I took up running. I read all that I could find on the subject and followed the advice of experts. Within three months I was able to run six miles without stopping. I could not believe it. I never thought it was possible for this forty-two year old, unathletic woman to do such a thing. But I did it and am so very glad that I did.

Running probably saved my life. My sense of well being increased steadily. My weight stabilized, I threw away my anti-depressant pills. I went back to work in nursing, this time as an instructor in the local vocational school. I taught high school students. I loved my job. I learned how to speak my truth. My life changed forever.

As I got stronger my marriage changed too. It was not easy for my husband to accept the more assertive wife I became. He made a valiant effort and supported my desire to go back to school for my baccalaureate in nursing. We moved to a bigger city. I went to college and he tried to establish his business in the more competitive climate of a larger community. He lost the mother I had been to him all those years. Things got worse and worse for us financially. His self-esteem went downhill as mine got better. When I graduated and got a good job as a head nurse, it was as though he did not have to pretend anymore. He did not want to stay married and after twenty-five years and four grown children, we separated. Through all the pain I continued to run.

I did not want it to be over, but it was. He went his way and I went mine. This time I did not experience the despair that my last "failure" had caused me. My running was my stress management tool as I grieved over the death of my marriage. I was from an era and an area where divorce was not really acceptable. I was ashamed to be seen in public without my wedding rings. In many ways, though, my divorce was a wonderful thing. My former husband is happy and healthy and after two open-heart surgeries that is a real miracle. Our children have survived the trauma; we are all a lot stronger. We love and support one another.

Running made all the difference for me. Any regular aerobic exercise will do the same thing. My only regret is that I did not start an exercise program sooner. If I do not live one hour longer than my allotted three score years and ten, as the result to my commitment to high level wellness, it does not matter. The truth is that the quality of my life is so much better now than it ever was before. Indeed, my life is one of great personal peace and joy. I realize now that I am entitled to abundance in every area and if there is a lack anywhere it is I who am responsible for that lack. Of course, there are challenges and problems. Life would be boring otherwise. But along the way I learned the wonders of wellness. How good it is to be fit and happy!

Life can be a journey of delight, especially for those who are physically, emotionally and spiritually fit. I have come a long way from the days when I felt I was a victim and was powerless to change most of the problems I experienced. If I can change, anyone can. This is not to say that I have all the answers for others, but I do have them for myself. So do you. The joy is in the discovering, the learning, and the becoming.

WORKBOOK EXERCISE

End of Chapter One

Answer "Yes" or "No" to the following questions:

1. I am employed in one of the "helping" professions such as nursing, counseling, social work or the ministry:

2. I am a volunteer in several church or community organizations:

3. I am the parent of young children:

4. I am a single parent:

5. I often feel stressed and lonely:

6. I rarely give myself permission to just BE:

7. I am often unhappy about the way I look:

8. I often feel tired and hopeless about myself:

9. If other people would change, I would feel happier:

If you have answered "Yes" to three or more of the above questions you may be ready to make some changes in your life. If you feel good all the time, happy about your life, your relationships and your work, there is no need to continue. If not, please go on to the next chapter which interests you, read it carefully and then go to the exercises at the end.

FURTHER READING

In this and other chapters I've generally avoided the day-to-day responsibilities, working conditions and other technical details of the nursing profession.* For nurses and other health professionals, such subjects are already well known and thereby redundant; for the general reader, only of marginal interest. For those in search of further materials, a highly selective listing is provided below.

Clarke, Margaret. *Stress and Coping in the Nursing Profession.* (Chapman and Hall, 1990).

Heron, Echo. *Intensive Care: The Story of a Nurse.* (Atheneum, 1987).

Humphrey, James. *Stress in the Nursing Profession* (Charles Thomas, 1988).

Ivory-Bertram, Margaritte. *Nursing: One Woman's Effort to Succeed.* (Landfall Press, 1991).

Kraegel, Janet, and Kachoyeanos, Mary. *Just a Nurse, From Clinic to Hospital Ward, Battleground to Cancer Unit: The Hearts and Minds of Nurses Today* (Dutton, 1989).

McConnell, Edwina. *Burnout in the Nursing Profession: Coping Strategies, Causes and Costs.* (Mosby, 1982).

Smythe, Emily. *Surviving Nursing.* (Western Schools, 1990).

Wolf, Zane Robinson. *Nurses' Work: The Sacred and the Profane.* (University of Pennsylvania Press, 1988).

---

* It is perhaps useful to note that in the original draft of this book, there was a discarded first chapter which laid out the day in, day out responsibilities of the typical staff nurse in rather painful detail. My motivation for this was to provide credibility for myself, i.e., that I was up-to-date on the latest innovations and developments. In other words, the proof that I knew what I was talking about. It seems, however, that all the fuss was unnecessary. I later submitted the full manuscript to a trusted friend and mentor for reading and suggestions. She praised the content but said the opening chapter could be discarded for the reasons listed above: limited relevance for the layman and redundancy for the professional. The titles provided above are but a small fraction of the available literature, and are drawn exclusively from the nursing field. This is because my expertise and perspective is from this area. There are probably books and studies about stress and burnout in all the caregiving professions. Check with a librarian or look in the *Subject Guide to Books in Print* or, for articles, *Infotrac* and *Readers' Guide.*

Chapter 2: Running For Your Life and Other Pleasures

Thoughts on Physical Wellness

Our bodies are simply the physical expression of our consciousness.

– Shakti Gawain

It only takes one person to change your life — you.

– Ruth Casey

Those of us in service to others paradoxically are not so good at taking care of our own bodies. We often stretch ourselves to the limit, physically, mentally and spiritually. We nurture and encourage everyone around us but we do not give ourselves the love and devotion to which we are entitled. We say we are "fine," disregarding our own needs, until it is almost too late.

Let us begin to look at our bodies with love and compassion instead of disdain and disrespect. Florence Nightengale was so right when she described the human body as a temple. The trouble with helpers is that we think far more about the needs of others than we do about our own. We can consider various ways to enhance our own health.

If our goal is to be healthy, then we need to know what health is. The traditional idea of health as the absence of symptoms is a misconception we can let go of. We caregivers see the absence of disease or remission of it, but we *rarely* encounter people who are genuinely healthy.

The best description of wellness I have found comes from

the book *The Holistic Way to Health and Happiness* by Harold R. Bloomfield and Robert B. Kory. They describe the healthy person as one who possesses the following characteristics:

> **lack of symptoms or abnormal test results, trim and physically fit**
> **full of energy, vigorous, rarely tired**
> **free from minor complaints**
> **alert, able to concentrate, clear headed**
> **radiant, clear skin, glossy hair, sparkling eyes**
> **active and creative**
> **able to relax freely, free from worry and anxiety**
> **self assured, confident, optimistic,**
> **satisfied with their work and the direction of their lives.**

If you have most of the above characteristics, that is wonderful. Unfortunately, many health care professionals are so concerned about others - clients, patients, family and community - that they don't pay attention to their own needs. If you find discrepancies when you compare your own health status to the above, you may want to do some self-evaluation. Loving oneself begins with taking care of the body. That is basic.

Wellness is actually a continuum:

Physical	**Absence of**	**High Level**
Death	**Symptoms**	**Wellness**

As you can see, death is on the left and high level wellness on the far right. Most people find themselves in about the middle of the continuum: we are asymptomatic, but there is so much room for improvement. It makes perfect sense that as an individual moves further over on the scale toward high level wellness, she will feel and look better. It is logical that she will be more effective and happier in her work world. She will be more resistant and resilient to stress. Where do you fit on the scale?

It is clear to me now that for most of my life I was about in the middle, like almost everybody else. But today I can honestly say that I am in a state of high level wellness. It is a planned effort that begins with commitment to a regular exercise program. I chose running to begin my journey into loving my body. You can choose any aerobic exercise you wish. I have friends who are dedicated swimmers, hikers, walkers, cyclists and aerobic dancers. Each has upgraded her fitness dramatically by getting involved in a sport she loves. And it does not matter how old you are when you start. The benefits will come to you at any age.

The most important thing about the exercise you choose is that it must be vigorous enough to cause you to sweat and increase your heart rate. The activity must last for thirty minutes so that you will receive full benefit. Choose something that you really enjoy doing and that you can do with a minimum of effort. Make up your mind that this is a gift you are making to yourself. Commitment is everything! There is absolutely no doubt that if you commit to loving your body through getting fit, you will promote your health.

An exercise program has been the best single thing I have ever done for myself and I know it. There are many days when I really do not want to get out and exercise. There are days when my feet feel like lead and I swear that I have never run before, certainly not any distances worth mentioning. But those are the days when I really need to exercise. I come in refreshed and feel like a new person. It is a high that I never tire of.

Running is great for me, but it is not for everyone. You would probably do just as well with a vigorous walking program. There is something for everyone. One of the best aerobic dancers I ever met was a woman who weighed over two hundred pounds. The critical thing is that you do SOMETHING and you do it *regularly*, just like brushing your teeth.

It is important that you do your new exercise program on a daily basis until you get your body in good shape. At about three months, the habit should be well set and you can cut down to three times a week if you need to. If you take off for more than two weeks at a time, you may very well lose the fitness level you worked to attain. You can continue your daily program if you are creative. I once read that Dr. Joyce Brothers takes a jump rope along with her wherever she travels. No matter where she finds herself, or whatever the condition of the weather, she continues her fitness program by jumping rope for thirty minutes every day.

If you like to swim and have access only to a small pool, you can do what my friend Maggie does. She has a harness which her husband put together for her. It is a belt-like apparatus which attaches to the sides of her pool with ropes. She hooks herself up and sets the timer for thirty minutes to swim in place. Maggie needs a cane to get around, but can she swim!

Learn to use your body to do more. Park your car farther away from the door of the supermarket. Walk up flights of stairs rather than waiting for the elevator. When I first met Mary Ann, a fellow nurse, I wondered how this petite woman kept her slim figure with her healthy appetite. I discovered that she never used the elevator if she could help it. She worked on the fourth floor of the hospital and always used the stairs. The rest of us began to imitate her and at first it seemed tough, but once we got used to it, we really enjoyed it.

Go for a walk instead of watching TV. Get in touch with your body and use it. The sad truth is that most North American bodies *rust out* rather than wear out. I don't subscribe to the argument that you cannot get out and exer-

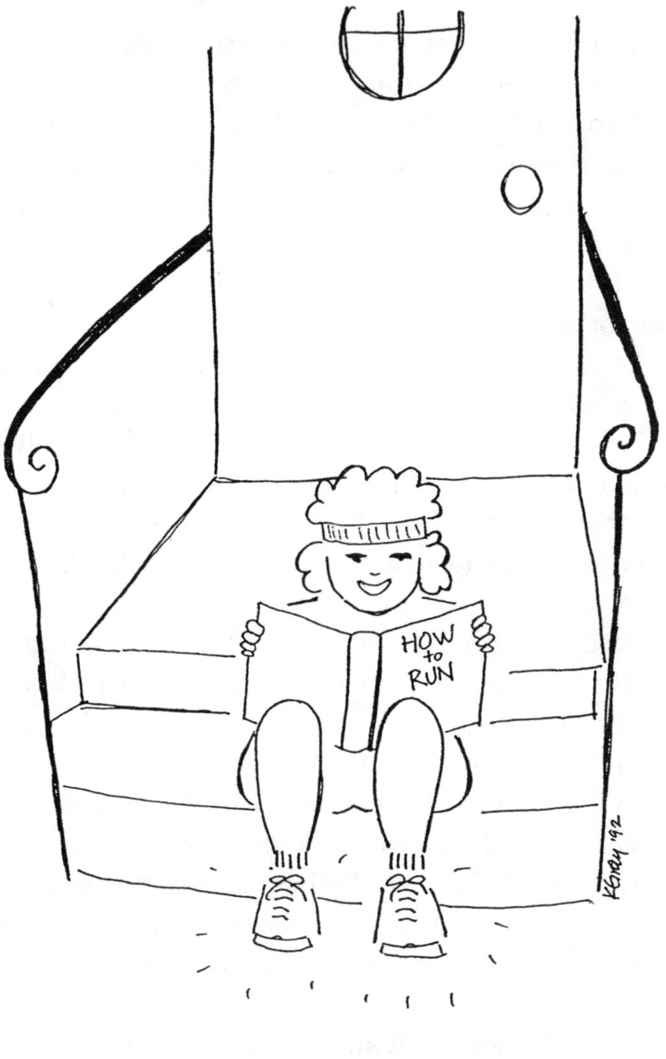
HOW to RUN
KGray '92

cise because you have been on your feet all day - the two activities are different. Exercise is refreshing and fun once you begin it.

The benefits of regular exercise are many and varied. The first thing that I noticed when I got fit was that I felt stronger. My endurance for physical work dramatically improved and I was able to work hard for many hours at a time without getting overtired. Then I noticed my resting heart rate had dropped from about eighty beats a minute to about sixty. My running really did make a difference. Today I rarely feel tired.

Once you commit to a regular exercise program you will begin to see some rewards. You will sleep much better and probably require fewer hours of sleep. Even when you eat enthusiastically, you will probably find that you are gradually losing inches of fat. You will build muscle tissue (which weighs more) and lose fatty tissue. That will make you look and feel slimmer, though your weight may stay the same. Exercising out of doors will give you the added benefit of being able to notice the beauty of the world around you. As you run or walk, you will begin to focus away from your problems or negativity and far more on the important issues of your life.

I don't know how it works with other aerobic exercises but I know that running will help you to become more creative. After you have been running for thirty minutes or so the brain will shift from the left side, the logical mode, to the right side, the creative one. When I first noticed this I was fascinated. When I got home I had to write down all my ideas immediately so that I could remember them. Later I discovered that the phenomenon is not uncommon among runners.

The most important time to exercise is when you've had a tough day at work, in other words, the days you least want to get out and be active. But these are also the days when your mental and physical health demand that you nurture yourself with a good workout. I call this decompression time and it works wonderfully for me. By the time I get back home, I have replaced my anxiety and disappointments with optimism and contentment.

One exercise benefit is that the body produces natural endorphins, the body's in-house pain killers and a natural soothing agent. When we produce our own, we are less likely to seek solace in food, alcohol or addictive behaviors of other kinds. Dramatic evidence of the amazing benefits of a regular program of aerobic exercise was found in a recent study. A group of older men was given a "growth hormone" to see if it would produce a sort of return to youthfulness. It did. Far more interesting was that the same results were achieved in a similar group of men who simply took up *regular aerobic exercise.*

Once you have made a commitment to you own physical activity program, stick to it. Don't let the weather or circumstances deter you. If you live in a place where winter limits your activity, find a gym or large building of some kind and work out there. It doesn't have to cost anything. I ran laps in the National Guard Armory in the little town where I lived.

You will meet the most interesting new friends when you start your program. They are the ones who are full of energy and life. Elizabeth is a teacher and counselor that I met while out running. When I met her, she had just returned from having spent five years teaching in Peru. Kathy is a geriatric nurse practitioner whom I met while out running, too. We have shared many wonderful hours while running or walking, and they have blessed my life in countless ways. The time speeds by when you have a friend to talk to as you jog or walk along.

It takes time to develop your fitness level, but according to health columnist Art Mollen, the investment is worth it:

If you are willing to pay a price, not in dollars, but in commitment, health can be obtained. The commitment is to your physical and mental well-being, and it is measured in time, patience, persistence and nurturing. Just as other investments grow in value, so will your investment in your health. It will be the best investment of your life.

WORKBOOK EXERCISE

End of Chapter Two

Health Assessment. Answer "Yes" or "No" to the following questions:

1. I have no symptoms of physical or emotional illness:

2. I am within ten pounds of my ideal body weight:

3. I am fit, vigorous and rarely tired:

4. I have no minor complaints:

5. I am alert, able to concentrate and clear-headed:

6. I look radiant, with clear skin, glossy hair and sparkling eyes:

7. I am active and creative:

8. I am able to relax easily:

9. I am free of worry and anxiety:

10. I am self-assured, confident and optimistic:

11. I am satisfied with my work and the direction of my life:

If you answered "Yes" to all the above questions, Hooray for you! You don't need this book! Please pass it on to someone else.

If you answered "No" to three or more of the above questions, please choose the exercise you would *most enjoy* doing. Suggestions:

running walking swimming bicycling jumping rope aerobic dancing

1. Commit to a regular program of exercise which brings you joy.
2. Start slowly. Pay attention to your body's needs.
3. Choose a time which is best and stick to it.
4. Do your chosen exercise every day for one month.
5. Re-evaluate your health status using the assessment questions.
6. Commit to exercising at least three times a week for the rest of your life.

There, don't you feel better?

FURTHER READING

Boston Women's Health Book Collective. *The New Our Bodies Ourselves.* (Simon & Schuster, 1992). The first edition of this classic work appeared in the 1970s and has become a solid resource on matters of women's health.

Diamond, Harvey and Marilyn. *Fit for Life.* (Warner, 1985). Discussion of the authors' nutrition and exercise program based on natural hygiene and diet. Followed by *Fit for Life 2: Living Health.*

Fixx, James. *The Complete Book of Running.* (Random House, 1977). Answers basic questions on the how, why, and how much of running. Comments of particular interest directed to women and runners over 40. The companion volume is *The Second Book of Running.*

Hughes, Rebecca. *Walking for Health and Fitness.* (Consumer Guide, 1988).

Katz, Jane. *Swimming for Total Fitness: A Progressive Aerobic Program.* (Dolphin Books, 1981). Presents fundamentals of swimming. Useful to persons of all levels of swimming ability.

LeMond, Greg. *Greg LeMond's Complete Book of Bicycling.* (Putnam, 1987). Topics covered include: cycling technique; training; bicycle maintenance.

Sorenson, Jackie. *Jackie Sorenson's Aerobic Lifestyle Book.* (Poseidon Press, 1983).

Chapter 3: Body Heat and Food for Thought

Nutrition and the Body

Health is a precious thing....the only thing indeed that deserves to be pursued at the expense not only of time, sweat, labor, worldly goods, but of life itself; since without health, life becomes a burden and an affliction.

– Montaigne

How very often have I heard beautiful, well-proportioned women bemoaning their "fat" and discussing the various new and wonderful diets that promise to shed pounds overnight! I was once one of them. I know that over the course of my lifetime I have lost at least a thousand pounds, sometimes at genuine risk to my health. But the fat came back. It was not until I learned to truly love and nurture my body by eating sensibly and exercising regularly that I no longer had to worry about dieting.

The human body operates much like a finely tuned and intricate machine. Such a creation requires a certain commitment to regular care and maintenance. Just imagine for a moment that you are the proud owner of a brand new, shiny luxury car. You have worked many long hours to purchase this beautiful machine. It runs like a top and is a joy to drive. It performs beautifully and responds to anything you want it to do. Because you love and appreciate this wonderful new car, you do everything possible to take care of it. You put only top quality gasoline in it and you make sure that it has plenty of oil. You keep the tires filled. All the fluids are the correct ones and are maintained at proper levels. You keep it clean, polished and properly insured. You would not even remotely consider the idea of running your precious investment on diesel fuel just because it is cheaper. You would not try to set out on a long and arduous journey without any gas in the tank. There is no way you would travel across the desert without water in the cooling system or an air-conditioner which was in top working order.

Can the human body be any different? Feed it junk food or no food day after day and expect it to perform well under challenging circumstances? It is unrealistic and even dangerous to treat the body with such disregard. But many of us do exactly that. The fact is that the body comes with a built-in warranty for about thirty years of dependable performance no matter what. It can be abused and taken for granted in many ways and still do the job. It may break down on occasion with colds, flu or minor injuries. But for most people a relatively healthy body can be expected for the first thirty to fifty years of their lives *even with poor maintenance.* However, there are very few nutritionally careless folks who do not ultimately reap what they have sown. The body, unloved and uncared for, will ultimately break down.

The subject of human nutrition has received much attention in recent years. Paradoxically, many of us are malnourished, due to misinformation, disinformation or just plain ignorance; proper eating is something that most people seem to practice very poorly. Happily, there are many excellent sources for nutrition information. A few of them are listed at the end of this chapter. Of the various diet programs available, I have found that Weight Watchers is the most sensible approach to healthy eating. It is not a diet in the usual sense, but rather an eating program which teaches people how to eat the correct foods in the correct amounts.

There is one thing I would add to their program, however, and that is to refrain from using more than minimal amounts of caffeine and artificial sweeteners. Plain pure food and clean water must be the mainstay of a health-enhancing diet.

One excellent source of nutritional information is author Annemarie Colbin, who has written *Food and Healing* and other books. She discusses many little-known facts about food and nutrition. One factor she explains in detail is the relationship between food and moods. I had occasion to learn exactly what she meant when I gave up caffeine. I had a day of a miserable blue mood with an accompanying headache. Since I had already eliminated most meat, sugar and dairy products from my diet I had only one day of the discomfort and withdrawal from coffee, tea and colas. Clearly my mood had been affected by the coffee which had been a large part of my daily fluid intake.

Many foods affect mood and behavior. Sugar is habit-forming and causes excitement as well as irritability. Starches, dairy products, vegetables, meats, fruits and spices all affect moods in various ways. We must pay attention to the body's response to various foods and chemicals.

We are so fortunate to live where we have access to fresh foods from all over the earth, all year long. Our foods are comparatively cheap. This makes them available to virtually anyone who wants them. It is my belief that *investing in good quality foods* is far wiser than scrimping on groceries and paying out the money later in medical bills. Good bodies need good maintenance. We can choose much of our food intake in the form of fresh, pure vegetables and fruits. It makes good sense to me that by consuming raw plant foods we are taking in the life force of living plants. A large fresh green salad every day is a part of my regular menu. I use dark lettuce and add a variety of crunchy, colorful vegetables, some tofu, nuts and occasionally cheese, and top it off with a nice low-calorie dressing. Delicious!

Choose healthy whole grain breads and cereals. Avoid sugars, salts and fats. Use low cholesterol products. Read food labels carefully and avoid those which are full of hidden chemicals, salt and calories. Cut down on fried foods. When we switch to pure, healthy foods, things may taste different at first, but it's surprising how quickly the taste buds respond to good quality nutrition.

By all means have what you want, but don't binge. All things in moderation, as the saying goes. Go easy on red meats; in fact, go easy on proteins period. Most North Americans eat far more protein than is necessary or advisable. It is good to have a small amount of protein at each meal, rather than all of it in the evening. If we have a constant supply, rather than a large amount late in the day, we will produce a steady source of healing energy rather than a lot which will only be turned into fat and put into storage.

Never eat unless you are hungry; snacking is unnecessary. Recognize the cues your body accepts as hunger signals. Often we think we are hungry when sight, sound, smell or socializing tell us food is available. If we eat only in response to genuine hunger signals and then eat in moderation, we will never be overweight.

Which brings us to the much discussed matter of thinness. I believe that North American women have been brainwashed by the fashion and beauty industries. We are constantly being hit by images which say that thin is beautiful. I would like to change the message to read: "Healthy is beautiful!" It is interesting to contrast this with the equally valid belief in other times and cultures that fat - or at least well fed - was fashionable. We were not all designed to be the same body build even if we shared a common height. Instead of cursing our variations, why not glory in our differences and meet our own vision of what we think is attractive? To paraphrase Leo Buscaglia, there's no one who looks exactly like YOU, honey! And that's wonderful.

I have learned how to accept and love my body as a unique and perfect creation of God. It does not meet Hollywood standards and never has. For most of my life I complained about my large hips. I wished that my breasts were larger and

I was miserable because I had ugly varicose veins. Certainly my little round tummy did not please me. I attacked my body every time I looked in the mirror. Poor body! It is amazing that it functioned at all the way I treated it.

Today I make a practice of giving my body positive affirmations and thanks every single day. When I am in the shower, as I soap each part of my body, I say, "Thank you for being so healthy and strong. Thank you for working so perfectly for me!" I look in the mirror and say nice things to myself like, "You're looking great today" and "You're my best friend." And, you know, I have come to believe it. My breasts are still small but they are healthy, and the nice thing about small is that they don't sag. My hips are still big but not too big. I still have varicose veins, in fact, I have even more. I wear a bikini when I go to the beach. Why not? I figure that if other people can't stand to look at this middle aged, imperfectly proportioned body in all its uniqueness, then they can look the other way.

I recall what Alan Cohen says:

Approval by others may bring encouragement but acceptance by myself brings freedom.

We are now seeing larger women who are assertive about their right to be themselves. I believe they are much better off staying at a stable weight than if they yo-yo themselves through a string of fasts and binges. As long as they *feel good* and *like themselves* who cares what the fashion industry or magazine ads say?

Remember the luxury car? Would we speed as fast as we could and then idle it as slowly as possible driving it around? What would happen to the engine? Why not run it at a nice steady pace all the time? It would be a lot better for the motor. The human body is much like any piece of machinery. Its running is the metabolic rate at which it uses its fuel. It really makes no sense to starve and binge and confuse the body.

When we starve, the body says, "O.K., I'd better conserve energy. Who knows how long the siege will last?" It then settles down to burn its food at a much slower rate. The body is very efficient. Then, when we eat normally again or overeat, it takes a while for the metabolic rate to get up to normal. Hence the rapid weight gain which occurs after a starvation diet.

So, be nice to the body. Feed it properly and it will look and feel better than you ever thought possible. No more grabbing a sugar-filled or even diet soda along with a salt encrusted bunch of potato chips for lunch. By the way, don't skip lunch no matter how important your work is to you. And don't forget to drink plenty of fresh, pure water every day. The human body is mainly composed of water. It must be refreshed, cleansed and cared for by having a steady supply. All the organs function a whole lot better if they are not forced to run dry.

There was a time when I suffered from premenstrual syndrome with its vicious and debilitating mood swings. I found that when I took a multivitamin tablet which was high in B and C the anger and lows disappeared and my emotional equilibrium stabilized. Many women who struggle with PMS have discovered that the same is true for them. At this time in my life I find it unnecessary to add vitamins or medication to my daily regime. My diet is exceedingly healthy and I no longer use any kind of mood-altering chemicals. That makes a tremendous difference in how my body functions. Good healthy food is the mainstay of my nutritional wellness today. I have learned what it is like to live in a strong and vibrant body and I have no desire to spoil that by using any chemicals.

We all have many choices every day, but *taking care of ourselves* is the first step. *A Course in Miracles* tells us that illness is the result of using the body lovelessly. I have seen the truth of this statement over a lifetime of caring for the sick.

WORKBOOK EXERCISE

End of Chapter Three

Answer "Yes" or "No" to the following questions:

1. I eat a well balanced diet every day:
2. I rarely choose red meats to eat:
3. I never add salt to my table foods:
4. I rarely eat fried foods:
5. I eat fast foods less than once a week:
6. I drink at least one quart of water daily:
7. I love and appreciate my body:
8. I never do crash diets:
9. I speak kindly to my body:
10. I never skip meals:

If you answered "Yes" to all the above questions you don't need this chapter. Congratulations! If you answered "No" to more than three questions you may wish to change some behaviors.

Choose three ways to commit to loving your body from the above list. Take the easiest behavior changes first. Each statement is a positive affirmation. Read them frequently.

Post the list where you will see it often. Do it. You will begin to notice an improvement in how you feel about your body within a matter of days. Good job!

From now on I will love my body in the following ways:

1. ____

2. ____

3. ____

FURTHER READING

Chopra, Deepak. *Perfect Health.* (Harmony Books, 1990). A physician trained in the traditional medical model combines Eastern and Western medical philosophies in order to establish the body's natural balance and reconnect mind and body.

Colbin, Annemarie. *Food and Healing.* (Ballantine, 1986). One of the most insightful books on nutrition, *Food and Healing* considers the subject from a variety of perspectives and traditions. The subtitle tells us much of the book's content: "How what you eat determines your health, your well-being and the quality of your life". The author's other writings include *The Natural Gourmet* and *The Book of Whole Meals.*

Dutton, James Scala. *Principles for Longevity: Eating Right for a Long Life.* (New American Library, 1992). Timely volume shows that good nutrition is necessary for quality life at any age.

Haas, Robert. *Eat to Win: The Sports Nutrition Bible.* (Signet, 1985). Concisely written book based on scientific research about nutrition as opposed to folklore about foods. Useful not only for athletes but for anyone who wants to be healthy.

Weight Watchers Fast and Fabulous Cookbook. (New American Library, 1984).

Weight Watchers New International Cookbook. (New American Library, 1985).

Chapter 4: On Not Worrying and Being Happy

Emotional Wellness

The bottom line is that I am responsible for my own well-being, my own happiness. The choices and decisions I make regarding my life directly influence the quality of my days.

– Kathleen Andrus

A complete reevaluation takes place in your physical and mental being when you've laughed and had some fun.

– Catherine Ponder

It really is a big ego trip to think that any of us, as an individual, is totally indispensable. I suspect that a lot of that kind of thinking has to do with the feeling that we must be in control all the time. If we take a sick day or even time out for lunch, the whole system would collapse, or so we would think. We have a hard time allowing a bit of chaos or unpredictability into our lives, especially our work lives, because we tend to be overly responsible. I observed this phenomenon in epidemic proportions in my three decades as a nurse.

The old truism that all work and no play makes Jane a dull girl is indeed true. All work also makes us prone to sickness and other forms of burnout. Lots of nurses and other caregivers have experienced it. I was able to return to my profession and take better care of myself. But so often we are tempted to simply abandon our professions. We cure the headache by cutting off the head.

Many of us have learned the joys and rewards of service to others, whether as volunteers or through our vocations. But it is important to take time for ourselves as well. We must not forget how to say NO. It is an *essential* step in the replenishment of our emotional resources.

One way of being more satisfied in our work situations is to make sure we take time for rest and play. It is not always an easy thing to do. I have worked with people who go through an entire shift without once sitting down for a break or a bite of food. Yet, a lunch break of only ten minutes, taken in a quiet place, is still a break. It would be nice, of course, if we could always count on thirty or sixty minutes away from the job. But if this is not the case for you, a few minutes taken by yourself is better than none at all.

What are you doing about your vacations? I personally think that workplaces need to give a lot more vacation time than they presently do. Management may have a different opinion. In any case, until that situation improves it is up to you to determine just how much time you need away. Holidays must be a chance for us to have a total change. And don't forget about sabbaticals. Three months. Six. Why not? Take that exotic trip you've been thinking about for years. To Asia. Or Europe. Sound nice?

When I feel the need, no matter where I am employed, I take an extended vacation. When I was working on a very busy unit in a large medical center in Hawaii I realized that I just had to take a month off. When I asked my superviser for the time she balked and we had to negotiate. Eventually I got what I wanted and needed. I was willing to state my needs and stand firm about getting them met. My boss wanted me to stay on her staff so she compromised. We both got something we wanted. My trip to the U.S. mainland was a great success and ultimately I was happier in my work.

No, we do not have to work all the time. We can say NO. It may seem scary or unfamiliar, but we can do it. Our work world will be the eventual winner by our setting limits on ourselves and exactly how much we can give to the system. Don't play the victim. To paraphrase Ann Landers, in a situation where someone is taking advantage of another, there is the one who is doing it and the one who is allowing it to be done to them. So speak up for yourself and what you need.

One of the most fascinating conversations I ever had with a nurse colleague was with Diane. She was a woman who had gone back to nursing school when she was past thirty. She told me that her first job as a new graduate was a painful but instructive experience for her. She was working in a situation where the pressure seemed overwhelming to her. When she complained about the unreasonable workload being placed on not only her but her peers as well, she was told that her *perception of reality* was wrong. She was informed that "the demands were the same everywhere." She was made to feel inferior because she protested.

She explained how she came to her awareness about what was going on in that institution: "I was on my way to attend a retreat for my twelve-step group and feeling very bad about having to lie in order to get the time off. I was emotional, frustrated and discouraged. I was turning the corner and looking over the ocean and it was almost like a light went on in my mind. I suddenly realized that these feelings were familiar because *I had felt them before* when I was enmeshed in an abusive relationship! I was doing the same things, trying to make it better, going overboard, trying to please my employer just the way I had tried to please my abusive spouse and I was still being made to feel that I would never measure up!"

As soon as Diane realized that her relationship with that particular employer was unhealthy for her and very unlikely to change, she decided to resign. She opted to work at a different institution where she quickly found out that things

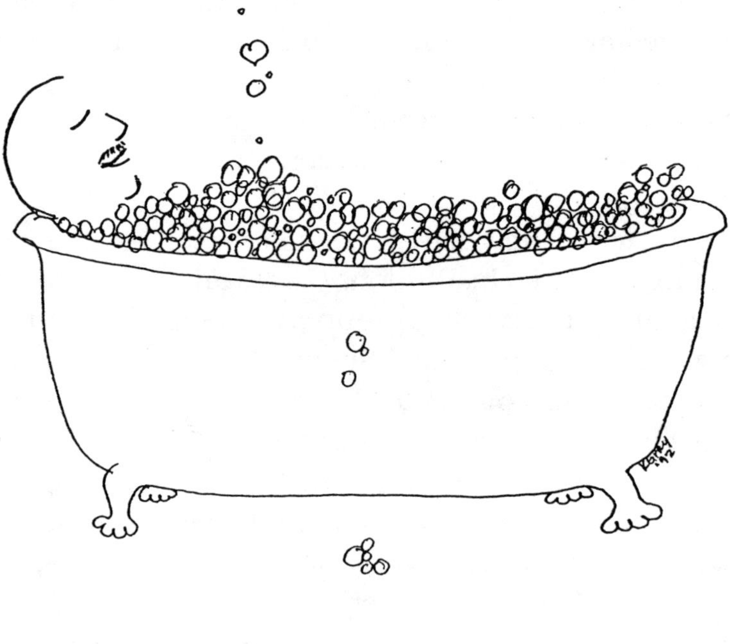

are not "that way everywhere." No longer was she willing to be isolated and controlled. Now she is in charge of her life and feeling very good about her assertiveness. This is one person who refused to be exploited. There are getting to be a lot more of us too!

One of the things I learned a few years ago was that I am a lot happier and much more productive when I work seventy-two hours or less in a work period rather than the traditional eighty. I can get along on less money but I cannot be as productive a worker when I am overtired. I have never had any trouble convincing my supervisors that this is a good plan. Every place where I have worked has been flexible about scheduling. If they are not, they soon find themselves losing staff to their competitors who know that if they are going to keep their staff happy (and indeed keep them on the job!) they must be sensitive to scheduling needs.

And what do we do on our days off? Do we lie out under a tree and just daydream? Do we go skating with the kids? Do we ride the carousel in the amusement park? Well, some of us do. We are learning how to love and nurture that little child within who probably never got enough play time during her growing up years. We *need to play* unselfconsciously, joyfully and frequently if we are going to be successful in our work. One thing you can do is make a list of the playful things that you enjoy. If you cannot find twenty-five different things to put on your list, it is probably time for you to take a look at your priorities in life. Once you complete your list, make sure you plan to do at least one joyful, playful, pleasant thing for yourself each and every day.

It may be a small thing, like soaking in a warm bubble bath for half an hour. It could be something which requires much more time, like hiking in the woods for a day, or sailing and surfing at a beach. Perhaps you would love to just curl up with a good book and put on some relaxing music and just be quiet for an hour or so. Maybe you need to go to the park and ride on the slide or the swings. Don't be self-conscious about your play time. Chances are that when people see you out flying your kite or blowing soap bubbles, they will have a sense of wistful wonder at the thought of perhaps allowing themselves a little play time someday. By all means, go out and play! If you just can't bring yourself to play alone, and you can't find a friend to join you, why not find a child who would like to have an adventure? Ask the child for suggestions. Children are great at thinking up fun things to do. We can be kids again. It's amazing how much better we feel when we include some play time each day.

There is really no good reason why we cannot have a little play at work too. The very best places I have ever worked are those which promote a pleasant, playful loving atmosphere for their staff. If the boss had a good sense of humor and is not rigid, chances are her staff members have a good time working together no matter how heavy the work load. I have had the most fun working in some of the most difficult and challenging units simply because the staff members express their love of life right there on the job. Hugging our colleagues when we greet one another after a few days off promotes a genuinely loving and supportive atmosphere for all. Having get-togethers away from work from time to time promotes cohesiveness. Life is meant to be enjoyed. We spend so much time at work; shouldn't it be a pleasant place to be?

If you presently work in a place which seems to be overly intense, with a lot of drudgery, complaining and unhappiness, I have a suggestion. Make your light shine there. Remember the saying, "It is better to light one small candle than to curse the darkness"? You will be surprised how quickly others respond to your refusal to be negative and promote real optimism instead. It works miracles in the most dreary situations.

We need to feel accepted and nurtured where we work. Life is much too short to endure misery there. If you have genuinely tried to make things better and nothing seems to be changing, why not get together with a group of staff people and your boss to problem-solve about it. Offer some suggestions. It may be easier than you think to improve things. Perhaps you need an outside professional to come in and evaluate the situation. Obviously not all work units have the same chemistry or morale level, but if all else fails you can always transfer to another section. If you cannot find the right spot in your institution, no problem. Look somewhere else. If you are a well educated, capable professional, there are many choices out there for you. You need only be open to the possibilities and let go of fear of change.

Rather than suffering in silence as a caregiver who gets less than enough care for herself, and then, in a fit of frustration and anger, simply drops out all together, take steps to remain in your chosen profession. We all have so much to offer. It really is a shame to waste all that compassion, caring and dedication by working in an area which does not use your education and talents.

Frustrating as jobs may be at times, in truth they are not the only source of our problems. It is easy to blame the job without looking at how we handle stress at home. Caregivers are often afflicted with control issues. That means we often find it easier to do it ourselves than to delegate responsibility for household chores to our mate or children. We are good at setting ourselves up for the abuse and overload at home as well.

We must remember that even though we are talented and energetic we cannot, indeed we must not, take total charge of the care of the home and family as well as our jobs. We must learn to set limits on our willingness to give physically, mentally and spiritually at home as well as at work. We must listen to our bodies. We can develop a team approach to the care of home and family. It does not make sense that we work very hard for ten or twelve hours and then come home and do everything for everyone else in our lives. If we think that caregiving is the cause of our burnout, we might want to look more closely at our living situation. Very likely, our habit of doing too much for others at work is repeated in our whole lifestyle.

The happiest nurses I've known have well balanced work and play cycles. They also have a lot of variety in their play time activities. Suzie is a great example of the well adjusted RN. She works hard in her job as a psychiatric nurse, but she plays regularly too. When I first met her, she was just learning how to scuba dive. She became so fascinated with the sport that she mastered it. She is now certified in ocean rescue. We all enjoyed her stories about the ocean and all of the new things she was learning as she played beneath its surface. I just ran into her again recently and she has taken up flying. She is well on her way to earning her pilot's license. I understand why she remains happy in her sometimes frustrating work. She doesn't work twenty-four hours a day. When work is over she goes out to play.

I know for a fact that Suzie has endured some painful times on the job, but she has such a buoyant spirit that the tough times did not get her down. She could always smile and see the bright side of everything. Some of her positive attitude is just her personality. She is a happy, loving person. But a lot of what keeps her going is her healthy play time and the many interests outside of work which nurture her soul. I suspect that Suzie will never burn out in nursing. I doubt that she will experience the kind of despair that drives so many young nurses out of the field forever.

One of the happiest caregivers I ever worked with was a beautiful Hawaiian/Chinese woman who took such good care of herself that she looked many years younger than her age. The first time I saw her, she came to our unit wearing a flower behind one ear in the Hawaiian fashion. I later learned that she spent lots of her spare time training for triathlons. She competed regularly and performed well. She not only managed a growing family as a single parent but somehow also found time to study traditional hula as well. Such a role model she is!

Leisure time activities are so critical to maintaining our mental wellness. There are an infinite variety of choices. One very contented psychologist I met has gotten immense satisfaction out of raising and training championship dogs. Another nurse does several different crafts. One is a gourmet cook who is always who is always learning about and expanding his culinary efforts. Roger is one of the most talented and capable nurses I know. He is caring and sensitive - sometimes he gets emotionally weary with the demands of his career. He gets great pleasure out of his hobby of carpentry. I suspect that he releases a good deal of tension by pounding and hammering away at his various building projects.

As a general rule, I've found that it is not a good idea for caregivers to do a lot of activities which are similar to what we do in our regular work. If the only recreational activity we have is built around service, we are in real danger of overload. I knew one social worker who realized that she had to stop her involvement with the crisis hotline in her community. It had started as an opportunity to get out of the house and meet some new people. But the work was too much like what she did all day at the hospital, and she realized she could not continue with it. Instead, she began to take art classes at the local community college.

There are so many interesting classes available, and many of them are free. One young nurse I know got immersed in studying Asian cultures. Even though she did not get off her evening shift until midnight, she was eager to get up the next morning and learn about the Orient. She worked hard at her job, but when she left work she changed gears and refreshed herself in a totally different way.

Why not take up learning a different language? How about quilting, sewing or knitting? Did you ever want to learn how to sky dive? I don't myself but I have friends who got a lot of pleasure out of it. What about gourmet cooking? When I lived in that small rural community in the Midwest, my friends and I complained about a lack of social activities. So we started a gourmet supper club. We discovered the cuisines of many foreign cultures. We also got together a larger group of women and began a fine arts club which promoted cultural activities such as our annual art show. We even arranged for a symphony orchestra to come for a performance.

You can travel all over the world in your imagination if you are an avid reader. The world of books can be a totally absorbing way to relax after a difficult day at work. Open up the pages of a good story and you are soon free of the nagging little thoughts which interfere with your time off. I love to read and for me one of the most effective ways to discover new books was to talk to a Lee, a nurse colleague. She read voraciously and we had similar taste in books. If I was ready for a good read, I simply asked what books she had discovered lately. We had some great discussions about literature. While we're talking about books, don't forget that most of the titles referred to in this book, and many, many more, are as close as your local public or academic library. If the particular title you want is not on the shelf or in the collection, ask the friendly reference librarian. They love to help.

Sometimes the reading leads to traveling in the more literal sense. My friend Joyce's reading stimulated her interest in travel. She has been all the world over and is still dreaming up interesting adventures. Listening to her talk about her trips to Egypt, Australia, Europe and all over the United States makes us all curious and eager to follow in her footsteps. Her eyes sparkle when she talks about the places she has been and the things she has seen.

Until I met Sister Richard Marie, I had never known a nurse who had worked full-time in the field for more than fifty years. For nearly thirty years she has been working with the Hansen's disease patients in Hawaii. She works forty hours a week in charge of the dressing clinic in the Kalaupapa Hospital. When things get too stressful for her, she goes fishing. It is quite a sight to see this amazing lady dressed in her full nun's habit, standing out by the surf with her fishing pole. Sometimes she is out there all day by herself and she always comes back to work with a twinkle in her bright blue eyes and a spring in her step. What a role model for graceful aging and happy nursing!

My favorite recreational activity is hiking. Nothing takes my mind off work like being outdoors. There are lots of hiking clubs around. The Sierra Club has numerous outdoor activities which also promote care of Mother Earth. Do things that bring you joy. If you have never attended a symphony or opera performance, don't wait, do it now. Live theater is accessible to anyone who lives in a city. Many rural communities have developed amateur theater organizations to meet their need for cultural diversity. Movies are an art form which are available anywhere, now that we have home videos.

Whatever the form our activity takes, it is important to remember that we must be DOERS as well as watchers. So many things that we do in our culture are spectator sports. While they have their place, it is important for us to be participants as well. We can get involved in athletic teams, card playing clubs or one of the many organizations for making music or saving the earth. No matter what responsibilities we have at home or at work, we can find time to do the things which are important. It is all a matter of setting priorities.

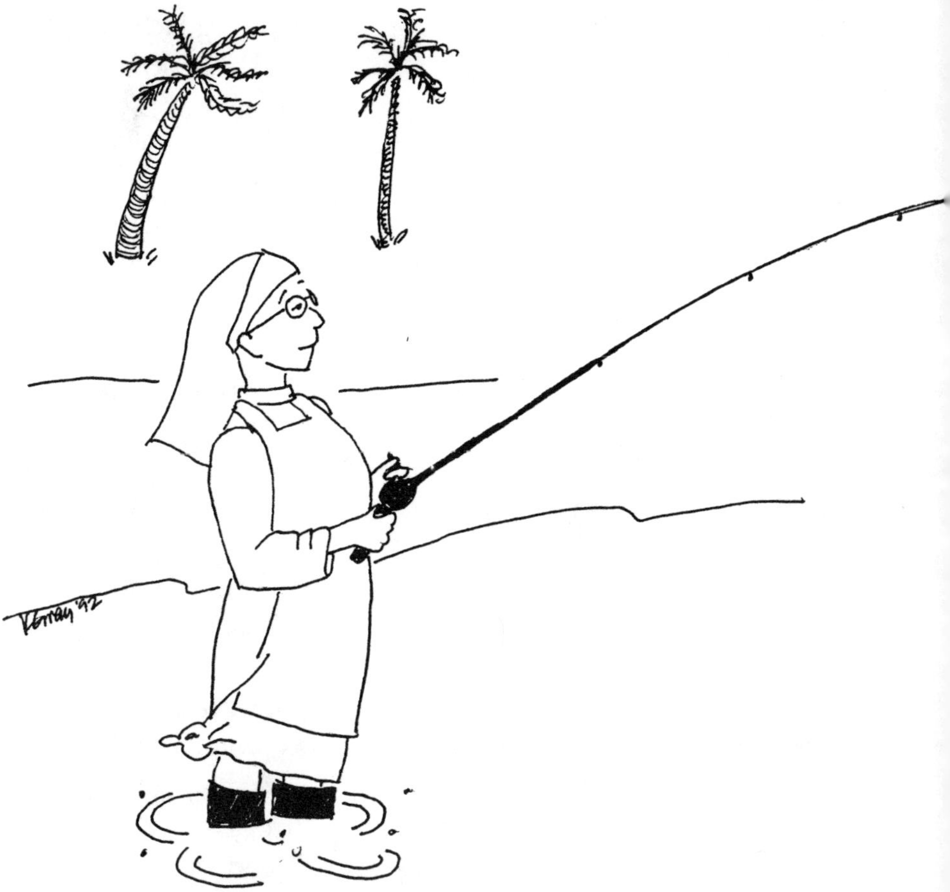
Kerrigan '92

One way to have a daily dose of play and fun is to find yourself a pet. Some of the happiest moments I've enjoyed in my life have been with animal friends. You can adopt a full grown dog or cat from the Humane Society or get a puppy or kitten very easily. Pets live *in the moment* and they give unconditional love. They can be wonderful friends and companions.

We need to spend time with other people in order to be happy, but we also need to spend time alone. It is important for us to learn to enjoy our own company. Surprisingly, few of us seem to like solitude, unless we are actively engaged in an activity or project. There was once a time when I too felt lost when I found myself alone. Today, I have learned to spend large amounts of time by myself and I never feel lonely. For me, that is a large evolutionary step on the journey of life. It has taken time to learn and practice this. I now treasure my solitary walks, my meditation out of doors and quiet evenings in my own company. Perhaps it is because I have learned to love myself and be at peace.

WORKBOOK EXERCISE

End of Chapter Four

Answer the following questions with a "Yes" or "No":

1. I refuse to spend my time worrying over things I cannot control:

2. Every day I schedule in time for some healthy play:

3. When I leave my job, I am able to stop thinking about it and enjoy the rest of my day, no matter what has gone on at work:

4. I regularly take part in social activities which I enjoy:

5. My friends include people who are not in the caregiving professions:

6. I spend at least half and hour each day outdoors:

7. At least once a month I invite friends into my home:

8. People describe me as a happy person:

9. If I am feeling exhausted and unhappy, I take a "mental health day" and spend the time in nurturing myself:

10. I laugh and play a lot:

If you answered "No" to three or more of the questions, please choose one of the following activities:

dancing - singing - a new craft - a new hobby - an interesting class - adopt a puppy - adopt a kitten - read a good book - join a club for social or exercise activity - plan a trip

Commit to your chosen activity and spend time each day in doing it, thinking about it and just loving it. At the end of one month add one more choice to your daily activities.

Doesn't that feel good? Do people tell you that you are more fun and more relaxed at work? Of course you are: you enjoy life and live it fully!

FURTHER READING

Benjamin, Carol Lee. *Second-Hand Dog: How to Turn Yours Into a First-Rate Pet*. (Howell Books, 1988). An excellent resource for people new to having dogs in their lives.

Borysenko, Jean. *Guilt is the Teacher, Love is the Lesson*. (Warner, 1990). Discusses the idea of guilt as the cause of disease and offers an alternative program of "spiritual optimism."

Gawain, Shakti. *Creative Visualization*. (Bantam, 1982). Meditations and exercises in which the imaginative power is tapped for self-transformation, based on the theory that we create our reality based on thinking patterns.

Kellogg, Terry, and Harrison, Marvel. *Finding Balance: Twelve Priorities for Interdependence and Joyful Living*. (Health Communications, 1991). How to learn to have a happier life through balancing activities. Includes an excellent reading list and appendix of sources.

Storr, Anthony. *Solitude: A Return to the Self* (Free Press, 1988). An interesting book on the subject of being alone and its relationship to the creative process.

Weiss, Daniel, and Chace, Susan. *Reader's Digest Crafts and Hobbies*. (Reader's Digest, 1979). Basic information for beginners of 37 popular crafts.

Chapter 5: Past Forgetting

Emotional History and Life Right Now

Super responsible people tend to be exploited. Somehow they almost demand it.

– Janet Geringer Woititz

Only those who dare truly live.

– Ruth P. Freedman

It seems to me that the majority of caregivers I have known (including myself) have come from dysfunctional families. The source of the dysfunction may be alcoholism, workaholism, a chronic illness in one of the members of the family, or any of a variety of other reasons. The caregiver may be unaware of the dysfunction, indeed may have to be for the situation to continue. I base my belief on observing many caregivers in clinical areas in several parts of the country. Just ask yourself or your peers* sometime what life at home was like. Ask if there was heavy use of alcohol or other chemicals. Ask if Mom or dad was chronically ill or unavailable.

Lest you get upset when you read these words just be open to the possibility that it may be true. Be completely honest in your assessment. If you are willing to do this, I am sure you will find at least one and perhaps many ways in which your family was dysfunctional. One of the problems is that it is difficult to look at the truth. It has been said that living with the alcoholic is like living in a home where there is an elephant in the living room. The only trouble is that we

---

* When using the word "peers" I refer generally to the health and caregiving professions, though the principle may apply to any profession.

all pretend the elephant is not there. Somehow it is just too scary or painful to confront the reality of living in such a situation. We usually ignore it and hope it will go away.

Descriptions of the healthy family and the dysfunctional family can be found in a variety of books. Typically, the healthy family is a safe place where each individual member is nurtured, supported and encouraged to grow in his or her own direction. There are no family secrets, no hidden agendas. There is consistent, open, honest communication. Children are shown respect. Adults behave as responsible citizens and the family interacts in a healthy, constructive way with neighbors, school and community. Each family member has his or her own circle of friends who are welcomed into the family home. No family member outranks any other in terms of value or importance. Children are raised to respect themselves and others. Discipline is administered honestly and fairly and is not intended to show the power of the parent or cause pain for the child. It is measured out carefully in a judicious effort to correct unacceptable behavior. In the healthy family there is no physical, sexual or emotional abuse of children or adults. The emotional needs of *all* family members are supported and met fairly and openly. The family and each of its members possesses a high level of physical, spiritual and emotional health. While family members may make themselves available to assist others in the larger community, they do not do so at the expense of their family commitment.

In a healthy family there is disagreement and conflict, but these are resolved with a minimum of anger and without rage. Children learn that anger is okay and that conflict is natural. Adults role model conflict resolution within the awareness of the children. All feelings are all right and there is a wide range of emotions. Children and adults both know that it is okay to feel things. They do not have to cover emotions or deny them; they do not have to take a pill or a drink in order to change their feelings. The family plays, works and lives together in a contented, satisfying way which meets the needs for nurturing of *every* member of the group.

It may well be that your family met all of the characteristics mentioned above. If that is so, you are very lucky indeed. My family possessed almost none of the above qualities. It has been my experience that most of the caregivers I have known came from families which were about as dysfunctional as mine was. The funny thing is that some of us grew up without realizing that the kind of behavior we saw being role-modeled by our parents was not healthy, supporting behavior. We thought it was normal. As a result of having been raised in dysfunctional families - whether or not the source of the dysfunction was alcoholism - we find that many caregivers possess most of the qualities of ACOAs (Adult Children of Alcoholics).

When I first read the characteristics of ACOAs, I was astonished and overwhelmed. Tears came to my eyes. I said to myself, "How can anyone know me so well?" But there it was in black and white, a list of many of my personal characteristics. Some of these qualities make us really good, loyal, conscientious employees, friends and family members, but some of them set us up for untold misery and frustration.

I had not known anything about ACOA's until my sister Judith shared her insights with me. She is a professional addictions counselor and had been at a regional conference on ACOA's. There she first read the list of ACOA characteristics as they are found in the pioneering work of Janet Geringer Woititz. She called me right after the conference where she had identified so much with all the traits discussed.

As we talked about our shared history we realized that although our parents were-meaning and responsible in their efforts, they did abuse alcohol in our presence on many occasions. She said she would send me a copy of the book and let me decide for myself.

Later I received Woititz's book, *Adult Children of Alcoholics*, in the mail. Judith had been so impressed by the work she had it autographed by the author. I devoured the book and suddenly things came into focus for me too. As a result of having read this book, I got involved in an ACOA support group which helped me get in touch with many of the things from my childhood and about my family that I had denied. I shared my experiences with people of all ages who were also in recovery from their painful childhoods.

One of the most difficult parts of this process was coming to an awareness that I had raised *my* four children in a dysfunctional family. The was a lot of shame and guilt in that emerging understanding. The dysfunction in my children's lives was different in many ways from what I had experienced as a child but nonetheless they had also been wounded. I could clearly see that I had seldom been emotionally supportive to my children and even now frequently disregarded their feelings. This was a form of emotional abuse and though it was not deliberate it was insensitive and demeaning to them.

I am deeply grateful for the work which has been done by such talented and dedicated professionals as Claudia Black, Rokelle Lerner, and John Bradshaw. Their contribution to my healing has changed my life in many ways. Furthermore it has impacted positively on such large numbers of people that the needs of children are addressed better today than they have ever been before.

Obviously alcohol is not the only drug which causes pain. There are countless addictions. There is the workaholic, the compulsive gambler, the sex addict, the relationship addict, the addicted runner, the compulsive shopper, the foodaholic, the bulimic, the anorexic, the nicotine addict, the hard drug addict, etc. When one member of the family is addicted to *anything*, there are consequences for every other member of the family. What is essential here is for us to see that addictive behavior on the part of parents directly impacts on the lives of the children. This is relatively new knowledge which has emerged in the past several years. Use of this information to understand ourselves better is very liberating.

Addiction separates us from others and it separates us from ourselves. When the parent is addicted to anything it causes him to be emotionally unavailable to the rest of the family. If the spouse of the addict happens to be a relationship addict, she is blind to the impact of the addict's behavior as it affects the children. The children then suffer a double bind. Not only are they living with the addict, but also with the codependent who enables the addictive behavior to continue. The codependent is often even less emotionally available to the children, preoccupied as she is with the behavior of the husband.

My daughter shared with me one of the things she could never understand when she was a child was the need to wait for "daddy to get home" before the rest of the hungry family could eat supper. At that time in my life I had a very romantic view of what the ideal family was like. I insisted on all of us sitting down together for supper even though my husband frequently was late getting home. I was often angry and resentful but it never occurred to me that we could eat without him. Thus, as in my case, dysfunction is passed from one generation to the next until we wake up and do something about it.

Many of us have grown up with a distorted view of what normal is. My response to having been raised in a very dysfunctional, violent family was to make sure there was no anger expressed in our home; it was just not acceptable behavior. During the twenty-five years that I was married I rarely *expressed* anger toward my spouse. I certainly was angry often, but we really never had a fight. Obviously that was just as unhealthy as was all the violence and unpredictability of living in my family of origin.

What I understand now is that we did not have anger in our house when I was growing up. We only had rage. It was sudden, shocking and terrifying, and I grew up fearing anger in myself and other people. Today I understand the dynamics of it and I am able to express and experience anger appropriately. I can allow others to be angry without turning into a quivering bowl of jello as I used to do.

In order to comprehend this distorted view of reality we need to look at the child as she perceives the world around her in her dysfunctional home. It is extraordinarily difficult for the child to trust her own view of reality when she is told that her perceptions are wrong. For example, the child comes in from play to hear screams of rage coming from her parents. Voices are harsh, and cruel obscenities are being hurled back and forth across the room. Naturally, the child perceives that something is wrong. She says, "Mom, Dad, what's wrong?" Mom's face is contorted in fury as she screams, "There is nothing wrong! What makes you think something is wrong?!" Dad curses and shrieks, "Get the hell out of here! You're always nosing around where you don't belong and causing trouble!"

So the little girl retreats in fear, pain and bewilderment. It has happened again. It must be her fault. There is obviously something wrong with her. Later when tempers have cooled, Mom and Dad may be extra sweet and nice to her in order to assuage their own guilt and pain. Again, the child is confused. She has been forgiven. Her parents do love her after all, in spite of what a *bad girl* she is. Aren't they wonderful? She is so grateful, and becomes more determined than ever to be a better person. She will be extra good. She will try even harder to please them. Maybe this won't happen again. But it does, over and over, Ultimately, she feels responsible for the problems. She becomes the super responsible, people pleaser.

This is how it happened in my life, and I suspect that many caregivers have had similar experiences. We tend to be overly conscientious, "I can take care of everything" types. We have a poor sense of our own boundaries and have a high tolerance for inappropriate behavior. We often have low self-esteem and seek validation from outside ourselves, unaware of our inherent worth as human beings. We accept the unacceptable. We try to please everyone around us. We almost always possess the characteristics of Adult Children of Alcoholics.

Unless we become aware of what is going on in our lives, we are very prone to burn out and leave our profession. We need to open our eyes and our hearts. We must learn how to nurture ourselves, take charge of our lives and *love ourselves enough* to be assertive about our needs. We need to take advantage of the support groups and written knowledge which are available to us. We can become the powerful, assertive women we can be who deserve to be treated well on the job and in all of our relationships.

One of the best things I ever did for myself was enroll in a workshop for Adult Children of Alcoholics. Along with eleven other adults of both sexes and all ages, over the course of ten weeks, I learned to take steps to self-acceptance. I faced the past squarely and became willing to forgive my family and myself for the harm that had been done. I learned to accept my humanity and my mistakes, and I began to learn how to love myself. Over the ensuing years I have continued to study and work the twelve-step program. I have been given freedom from the compulsion to be everything for everyone. I have learned how to set limits on my time. I can say "No" at work and at home. I can remain in my profession and be happy with it.

Never again will I allow myself to be exploited. I don't need to do that anymore. I understand very clearly now that when I take good care of myself I am far better equipped to be fully present for the people around me.

WORKBOOK EXERCISE

End of Chapter Five

Answer the following questions with a "Yes" or a "No":

1. My father was an alcoholic or addict, not in recovery:

2. My mother was an alcoholic or addict, not in recovery:

3. One of my parents could be described as workaholic, not in recovery:

4. One of my parents was chronically ill or absent from home:

5. I often felt confused and frightened as a child:

6. I was often punished physically as a child:

7. As a child I learned that in order to be appreciated I needed to be quiet and make few demands:

8. When I was afraid or insecure as a child, my parents ignored, derided or dismissed my concerns:

9. There was rage and/or violence in my home:

10. Leaving home as soon as possible was a goal for me when I was growing up:

If you answered "Yes" to any of the above questions you may have been damaged as a child. Your choice to become a professional caregiver may have been based on the assumption that you were "not good enough" just the way you were.

Choose one or more of the following affirmations. Print it out in large block letters and post it where you can see it during the day. Believe it!

1. I am whole, perfect and complete just the way I am.

2. I love and accept myself just the way I am.

3. My most important and reliable friend is ME.

4. I am entitled to be happy. I deserve joy in my life.

FURTHER READING

Beattie, Melody. *Codependents' Guide to the Twelve Steps.* (Prentice-Hall, 1990). The author shares her own experience in recovery.

Beattie, Melody. *The Language of Letting Go: Daily Meditations for Codependents.* (Harper/Hazelden, 1990). Assistance in letting go of self-defeating behavior.

Black, Claudia. *It Will Never Happen to Me.* (MAC, 1981). More helpful information on the subject of being raised in a home affected by addiction.

Bradshaw, John. *Bradshaw on the Family: A Revolutionary Way of Self Discovery.* (Health Communications, 1988). Bradshaw discusses the psychological effects of belonging to a dysfunctional family.

Bradshaw, John. *Healing the Shame That Binds.* (Health Communications, 1988). Recognizes problems people have who were raised in dysfunctional and alcoholic families and suggests methods for dealing with it in a healthy way. Similar issues are discussed in the author's *Homecoming: Reclaiming and Championing Your Inner Child.*

Davis, Laura, and Bass, Ellen. *The Courage to Heal: A Guide for Women Survivors of Child Sexual Abuse.* (Harper Collins 1988).

Lerner, Rokelle. *Daily Affirmations for Adult Children of Alcoholics.* (Health Communications, 1985). Daily inspiration for building healthy self-esteem.

Snow, Candace, and Willard, David. *I'm Dying to Take Care of You: Nurses and Codependence, Breaking the Cycle.* (Professional Counselor Books, 1989).

Steinem, Gloria. *Revolution from Within.* (Little, Brown, 1992). The author shares hopeful and uplifting stories of the emerging power of people who are overcoming negative scripts from childhood.

Whitfield, Charles L. *Co-dependence: Healing the Human Condition.* (Health Communications, 1991). A guide for achieving healthier, responsible behavior.

Woititz, Janet Geringer. *Adult Children of Alcoholics.* Revised edition. (Health Communications, 1983). A concise and informative explanation of the painful results of being raised in a dysfunctional family.

Chapter 6: Unhealthy Pleasures and Obsessions

Addictions and the Caregiver

My spiritual, mental and physical healing is a life-long investment of my time, my energy and my love.

– Rockelle Lerner

Create your life to be as beautiful and loving as you desire it to be. Know it is up to you.

–Terry Cole-Whittaker

An addiction is a compulsion, a loss of control, a craving for something. It comes from a need to avoid feeling; a fear of facing life head on without some kind of "drug" to make it easier to deal with reality. Almost anything can become an addiction from a drug to a behavior. The caregiver seems to be more vulnerable than many people to addictions of all kinds. Unfortunately, many caregivers seem unaware of their dependencies. Those of us who have become aware fill the rooms of twelve-step meetings across the country.

Why are we such compulsive folks anyway? Many of us learned early on how to cope with our environments by becoming super-responsible children. We did not learn how to play. We took life very seriously. Some of us did not even get to be children. Many caregivers I have known had full responsibility for families when they were just pre-teenagers. Many of us were emotionally, sexually or physically abused. We learned quickly how to be good little girls or boys, how to be quiet, how to ignore our own feelings and our own needs for nurturing. We became the nurturers - professional or otherwise.

We have carried with us a tendency to block out our feelings or to hide them in a variety of ways. Often we become hooked on various chemicals, perhaps not realizing at all that we're addicted. Through compulsive behavior we create the illusion that we don't have to deal with our feelings. We numb, ignore and deny the reality of what's going on inside. The only trouble is that the feelings don't go away. They become submerged and distant but they are still there. Sometimes they explode in very destructive ways. I have heard more than one caregiver say that she had seriously considered suicide as an option at some time in her life. It seems frightening to face our emotions but the only way around them is to move right through them; trying to pretend they don't exist does not make them go away.

There are such a variety of human feelings to be experienced and expressed. Often we have become so out of touch with them that we cannot even give them a name. I heard one caregiver say that most of her life she was aware of having only three feelings. They were fear, anger and joy. It had only been after her long association in twelve-step groups that she began to learn about the many nuances of emotions. The three primary feelings which she was able to recognize were so strong that she had to acknowledge them. The more subtle emotions were harder to identify and it took her much diligent effort to be able to recognize them.

When I emerged from the long marriage where I constantly ignored my own emotions and paid close attention only to the behavior and needs of people around me, I did not even know what I felt. I did not know who I was, or what I needed. Now I know that if I get an unexpected emotion I must go within and ask myself what is going on. What is it really which is making me feel so uncomfortable (or so good)? Only through introspection have I come to understand and accept all of my feelings. For years I tried to disown them. Today, I am very grateful for all of them. They add depth, interest, variety and perspective to my humanity.

As children in dysfunctional families, chronically deprived of nurturing, we learned early on how to feel better. We got good feedback from others when we covered up or denied our own needs and we began to serve the needs of the other people around us. I have met so many caregivers who were "little mothers" or surrogate wives in their families. We cooked, cleaned, baby sat, washed, ironed, and did numerous household tasks. And we were praised. That gave us comfort and a sense of being loved or appreciated. So we did it more. Often we supplanted the role of the mother because Mom was absent, in one sense or another. We tried so very hard to please. Often, though what we did was extraordinary, it was not acceptable to parents who had unrealistic expectations for children.

This making things better for others gradually became a habit, so we naturally gravitated into a field of work where this behavior was valued and rewarded. We found that patients gave us the appreciation which had often been denied us. That was a heady experience when it first happened to me. It still is. When patients and their families praise my efforts, I get a sense of great inner satisfaction. There is nothing wrong with that, but if outside validation is our only comfort, we are in for trouble. It is essential that our good feelings come from within ourselves. Outside strokes are nice, but they can be capricious and undependable.

Looking outside ourselves for things which make us feel good can easily lead us to looking for ways to fill up the inner void by using chemicals. Alcoholism is a trap for so many of us. That is not strange, since many of us came from alcoholic families. Not only have we learned unhealthy coping behaviors in the alcoholic home, but we are generally susceptible to the disease itself. Studies have found that children of alcoholics are much more prone than the rest of the population to becoming alcohol-dependent. That tendency is true for children who have been removed from the alcoholic home, just as well as those who are raised within it. It is a fact of life and we must be honest as we look at the possibility of addiction.

Our society foists drugs of all kinds upon us, with alcohol getting more than its share of hype. The media are full of advertisements for alcohol; any social situation is always an occasion to open up bottles. If we find ourselves using alcohol on a daily basis, no matter how much or what kind, we need to look at our behavior. If we find ourselves having a drink or two to unwind and get to sleep at night, alarm bells should ring us awake. Alcohol is one of the most widely used addictive drugs in Western culture, and caregivers are at risk, even more than the general population.

Caregivers frequently marry alcoholics or other types of addicts. It is much easier for us to worry about the needs and problems of others than to recognize and take care of our own needs. We perpetuate the unhealthy relationship. If our partner needs us then of course we'll feel important and powerful. We become part of a dysfunctional relationship. We continue the cycle by becoming codependent and/or addicted and then we produce more codependent and/or alcoholic offspring. It goes on for generations and will do so until we heal ourselves and break the pattern.

If you walk into any bookstore, you can quickly find the adult children of alcoholics. We are clustered around the self-help books. Whether or not we are aware of it, we have come to believe that fixing the rest of the world is our responsibility, much in the same way that we have taken on the belief that it is up to us to fix the family. We seem to think that if only *we* become better, more educated, more aware, we could be more helpful. It is a very good thing to get more knowledge, awareness and insight. But the first person to fix is oneself.

When we are tired, the natural and sensible thing to do is

slow down or rest. But often we cannot or will not take the time to do so. We choose to jolt our systems into continued activity when we are long past the need for a break. We get our jolt from coffee, colas and teas. They are all legal. And don't misunderstand. I enjoy a warm, rich cup of coffee as much as the next person, but like anything, used to excess it is harmful to the body and the psyche. It is not uncommon for many caregivers to be addicted to caffeine, given that we often have to stay awake and alert when our bodies yearn for the comfort of a warm, cozy bed. Caffeine revs up the body's motor and causes a great deal of unnecessary wear and tear on the human machine.

Sometimes we become drug addicts. I don't know what the statistics are on the number of caregivers who are addicts - it's anybody's guess. In hospitals, nurses have access to drugs of all kinds. If we really wanted to, we could find ways to steal and use whatever we wanted. And of course street drugs are available to anyone. I have met nurse addicts both on the job and in twelve-step meeting rooms. It is easy for nurses to get prescriptions for drugs from the many physicians who come onto our units each day. Some caregiver addicts don't get caught. Some lose their licenses. Some get help, but many do not.

The most addictive drug of all in nicotine. It takes less than a week to withdraw from hard drugs such as cocaine or heroin but it takes two to four months to withdraw from nicotine. This addiction affects many caregivers. It's indeed deadly, as we know all too well. We have seen the people who are dying of lung cancer and emphysema. We care for damaged bodies of those who have suffered serious circulatory disorders or lung damage as a result of smoking. One would think that having seen all of that we would vow never to smoke. But many of us do. It is virtually guaranteed that to continue smoking is to create serious health problems. We all have to let go of the notion that smoking is just a bad habit.

It is more like walking down the center of a railroad track when there is a train coming. Unless you get off the track, you will get hit by the train. You just don't know when it's going to happen.

There are twelve step groups for people who are determined to give up smoking. The people who have been most successful at letting go of their addiction to smoking have systematically applied the AA principles to their recovery from nicotine addiction. In my experience, the easiest and fastest way to quit smoking is to enlist the support of a certified clinical hypnotherapist who treats many people with this problem. Such therapists are available in any major city. Ask your friends who have used this method to refer you, or call your health care provider for a referral. The National Medical/Dental Hypnotherapy Headquarters* can also be contacted for information.

Finally, it is possible for caregivers to get hooked on our own adrenaline. We become addicted to the excitement of working in intensive care areas, emergency rooms, labor and delivery areas and other fast-paced, tense work environments. Some caregivers seem happiest when they are in crisis: rushing, managing, hurrying, racing, directing, doing, doing, doing. I'm the first to admit that I've experienced the highs of working in emergency rooms and intensive care units. I know how good it can feel. But I have seen caregivers burn out, myself included, who have simply done it far too long or failed to pace themselves. Adrenaline addiction is subtle and is highly rewarded in some professions. We often carry this addiction over into our personal lives. Crisis at work and crisis at home. An unhealthy situation all around. The crisis manager mode can assume strangely nuanced shadings. I know of one emergency room nurse who offered a friend some money to pay her rent. The friend declined and

* Address is listed in the Appendix.

later discovered that the nurse had had her own telephone turned off because she failed to pay her own bills.

Food addiction is not uncommon for caregivers; on every unit one will see at least one caregiver who is grossly overweight. She may represent only the tip of the iceberg. I've met several nurses who are bulimic. They binge and they purge; food is at the center of their coping mechanisms. If they get into a really uncomfortable place, they eat. They eat until they cannot eat anymore and they throw up and use laxatives to clean out the body, sometimes suffering horrendous health problems as a result.

Many of the caregivers I have known who have suffered from severe weight problems or eating disorders were sexually abused or molested as children. As these people became committed to their recovery from that trauma and pain they were then able to deal effectively with their problems with food addiction.

Anything can become an addiction. Some drugs or behaviors are simply more accessible, common or socially acceptable than others. Since we learned very early on how to get validation from outside ourselves, we often fall prey to relationship addiction and sex addiction. We learned to get gratitude and recognition by serving others. Often we mistook these feelings for love, and we try to fill up the emptiness by being physically involved with men. We can become addicted to sex or love. We can, as I did, make another human being our god and be addicted to the relationship.

Denial is one of the prime characteristics of addiction. In few other diseases is the person willing to risk her life to the point of death in order to hide the truth about herself from people who probably already suspect that she has a problem with alcohol or some other "drug." I know about denial. For years I questioned my drinking habits, but only to myself. I looked around at the way in which others abused alcohol and decided that I was no different than they were.

But there came a time in my life when I had to know the truth about myself and when I was told by a person whom I very much respect that I was "probably alcoholic." I had to accept the truth, and doing that has indeed set me free. When I went to my first AA meeting, I did not go happily. Rather it was with dogged determination to be as healthy as I could be in every area of my life. Interestingly, there were three other nurses, all about my age, at that meeting. I was surrounded by total and unconditional love for the first time in my life. I discovered later that none of those women regularly attended that particular meeting. As they say in the program, a coincidence is God working anonymously.

I can see now as I could see soon after I committed to a sober life that this was the missing part of the puzzle for me. I realize that I have health and power in as much as I am relentless about facing the truth and dealing with it. I am a "grateful alcoholic in recovery," as I have said in the meetings. I doubt I ever would have found true inner peace and happiness if I had continued to deny my "handicap." As an alcoholic I realize that I am much like people who have other kinds of handicaps. I cannot change the facts about my genetic make-up and limitations any more than any other person. It is in accepting the truth, facing it with courage and doing what must be done to move into recovery that I claim my power.

Many of us are susceptible to our addictions, and caregivers have no monopoly on obsessive behaviors. It must also be said that I've known many healthy, happy and well-adjusted caregivers and health professionals. But our society, with all its obvious merits and benefits, can be very seductive: we are constantly enticed by messages which say there is a quick fix for everything. So we tend to think that this is true, when certainly it is not. The real truth is that we must learn how to face our fears, whatever they are, and feel our feelings, no matter how frightening. We need to learn how to validate and love ourselves for the unique beings that we are. We all deserve a good life, filled with happiness, satisfaction and serenity. It will not come without some effort on our part and it will not happen overnight.

We must confront whatever it is that is holding us in a negative pattern. We need not do it alone; there is plenty of support available for us. We can nurture the little child within us who was never appropriately cared for. We can speak kindly and softly to her when she is afraid. We can reassure her that we will always be there for her and then do it. We need to be willing to grow and change, to let go of our addictions and really experience life fully. Ann Wilson Schaef expresses it thus:

There is no transformation without recovery, and there is no recovery without transformation.

WORKBOOK EXERCISE

End of Chapter Six

Answer the following questions with "Yes" or "No":

1. I use alcohol on a daily basis:

2. I use nicotine/marijuana or other mood-altering chemicals:

3. Tranquilizers or sleeping medication help me cope with the pressures of life:

4. Sometimes I drink so much alcohol I can't remember what I did during my drinking activities:

5. I often wish that I could stop drinking or using:

6. There have been times when I wanted to say NO to nicotine, alcohol, drugs, sex or food *but I just could not*:

7. The only way I can feel good or relaxed is to use food, cigarettes, sex, drugs or alcohol:

8. I have often wondered if I shouldn't cut down on my drinking:

9. One or both of my parents had a problem with drugs, smoking or alcohol:

10. I use exercise, television, food, drugs, sex, alcohol, nicotine, or religious fervor in order to avoid dealing with my pain:

If you answered "Yes" to one or more of these questions you may have a problem with addiction. Choose at least one of the following activities:

1. Make an appointment with a certified addiction counselor for an evaluation of your drinking/using activities. You can find the help you need by calling the office of an *accredited* Treatment Center in your area. They are listed in the Yellow Pages under "Drug Abuse and Addiction - Information and Treatment." Resolve to follow the advice you receive there.

2. Begin attending regular meetings (at least weekly) of a Twelve-Step Group which focuses on recovery from your particular addiction.

3. Commit to a life of sobriety. Enlist the support of a sponsor and follow her/his advice. You'll be glad you did.

FURTHER READING

Allison, Patricia. *Hooked - But Not Helpless: Ending Your Love/Hate Relationship With Nicotine.* (BridgeCity Books, 1990).

Arteburn, Stephen. *Addicted to Love.* (Servant Publications, 1991). Discusses recovering from unhealthy dependency in romance, relationship and sex.

Beattie, Melody. *Codependent No More.* (Hazelden Foundation, 1987). The primer for people whose "drug of choice" is another person.

Booth, Father Leo. *When God Becomes a Drug: Breaking the Chains of Religious Addiction and Abuse.* (Jeremy Tarcher, 1991). An examination of the phenomenon of religious addiction and abuse and offers a program of recovery based on the twelve steps.

Kasl, Charlotte Davis. *Women, Sex and Addiction.* (Ticknor & Fields, 1989). Description of how women find themselves in sexually addictive patterns. Extensive documentation.

Minrith, Frank and others. *Love Hunger: Recovery From Food Addiction.* (Thomas Nelson, 1990). Offers a complete weight-loss and maintenance program for compulsive overeaters, incorporating addiction counseling.

Norwood, Robin. *Women Who Love Too Much.* (Health Communications, 1985). Landmark examination of the codependent relationship as it relates to women and self-esteem.

Roth, Geneen. *When Food is Love.* (Plume, 1992). Explains the relationship between food and intimacy.

Waldrup, Heidi. *Showing Up for Life.* (Hazelden, 1990). A psychological portrayal of the author's triumph over her eating habits.

Chapter 7: Just Between Us

Finding Serenity in Twelve-Step Groups

God, grant me the serenity to accept the things I cannot change, the courage to change the things I can, and the wisdom to know the difference.

– Rheinhold Niebuhr (attr.)

Unless we are gelled and whole in our own consciousness, we are not in a position to serve.

– Alan Cohen

The grandfather of all the twelve-step groups is Alcoholics Anonymous. That organization came into being in a most surprising way more than fifty years ago. It continues to astound the world with its success. AA was started by two chronic and sick alcoholics. Bill W. and Dr. Bob had been very successful in their respective careers in business and medicine but they both had lost everything due to their inability to handle alcohol. They had tried every known cure for their addiction but nothing worked. In desperation they turned their will and their lives to God. They talked, shared, prayed and worked together and somehow, *by doing it together,* managed to stay sober. They began to spread the word to other alcoholics and found that their program worked. The rest, as they say, is history.

Together with other recovering alcoholics they wrote the book, *Alcoholics Anonymous,* lovingly called the "Big Book." It is indeed divinely inspired, for it holds the key to recovery to anyone who takes the time and effort to practice its principles.

These pioneers came to understand that the essence of humanity is the spiritual part of mankind. It is by numbing ourselves that we become lost and afraid. Only by honoring our higher selves, allowing the divine part within to lead us in every part of our daily lives, can we be fully human. We need to lead our lives with complete and rigorous honesty and we must understand that our greatest joy comes from expressing ourselves as the unique and wonderful beings we are.

It is the deep honest sharing and unconditional acceptance of each member which create the powerful bonds of love and support in AA. Today, there are twelve-step programs for people with many different kinds of problems. Overeaters Anonymous, Gamblers Anonymous, Narcotics Anonymous, Sex-Addicts Anonymous groups all provide the means for persons with various types of addictions to learn new and healthy coping behaviors. As was pointed out in the previous chapter, ours can be a very addictive society, but help is readily available for anyone who has a desire to change and grow. The yellow pages of any telephone directory will list the various organizations which are out there. If there is no group in your town, start one. That is what folks all over the world have done. Write to the national headquarters of a specific group for information and get going.* You will not be alone for long.

It is more liberating than one might expect to find yourself in a group of loving, supportive people who really understand where you are coming from. Suddenly, you are not alone anymore. No matter what you share in the group meeting, it has been said before. There is nothing too shocking, too unacceptable to be told. What a relief it is to put down the burden of dealing with life without the proper tools!

---

* Addresses listed in the Appendix.

Today, I am committed to my twelve-step program. I live my life as closely as possible to the precepts in that program. I learned that "we are only as sick as the secrets we keep." I am now completely willing to share who I really am with the members of my groups. These meetings can be among the most powerful experiences in human communication because of the trust and support which is always present in the fellowship. No one is excluded; no feeling is too bad to express. What we do is share our "experience, strength and hope" with each other.

I once heard Dr. Bernie Siegel explain the importance of peer support. He is a well-known oncologist* and surgeon who has pioneered support groups and self-healing for people with life-threatening illness. He suggests that we get into a support group of any kind; that everyone needs a place where she can be fully accepted and supported in life. He further advises that if you don't meet all the technical qualifications for a twelve-step group, go anyway. But get into one.

It is indeed true: our lives take on a new dimension and we become more self-accepting, accepting of others and more serene than we have ever been in our lives. We learn to become healthier by working with others as sponsors and friends.

If we are using alcohol, drugs, food, sex or anything else to cope with the pressures of our lives as caregivers, then we need to take a critical look at our behavior. We must understand that just stopping an unhealthy coping process is not the whole and final answer. In AA they say, "If you stop drinking and don't work the program you're still a drunk. You're just a dry drunk." And that is very true. It is just as true with the other addictions. Stopping will just remove your source of numbing and stress relief, but in the process this may cause even more problems than before.

---

* *Oncologist*: a physician who specializes in tumors.

I knew a woman who was a perfect illustration of this point. She is an enormously talented and attractive person. She was one of the flower children of the 1960s. She became addicted at alcohol and hard drugs during that time. For many years her life was ruled by those addictions. She saw that she was headed down the path of complete self-destruction, so she gave up both of her addictions. She did not join a support group, she did not work the twelve steps, and she did not get a sponsor. Before very long she had replaced her two previous addictions with two new ones, food and religion. Now she weighs over three hundred pounds and spends most of her time on church activities.

She is still escaping from a reality which is too painful for her to deal with without her "drugs". She is unwilling to use the tools which are readily available to her in order to live a sober, healthy life. She exchanged two addictions which she saw as being evil and threatening. But she is still a slave. She is unlikely to find true serenity until she is willing to face her fears honestly and deal with them.

It was once said that no one could help the alcoholic until he hit bottom, realized it and asked for help. Not true. It is possible to intervene, often very successfully when professional help is sought in order to do so. A well-known example is Betty Ford, a woman of courage and honesty who has shared the truth about her dependence on drugs and alcohol. Her family, in desperation, sought professional help for her. Together they worked with a qualified addiction counselor who orchestrated what is known as an intervention. In this process, the alcoholic or user is confronted with the truth about her drinking or other addictive behavior and how it has impacted on the lives of the loved ones. This is done only when the impaired person is fully sober and the family is prepared with alternatives for treatment. It is a serious process and can be life-changing for everyone concerned. An accredited addiction center can give you information on how

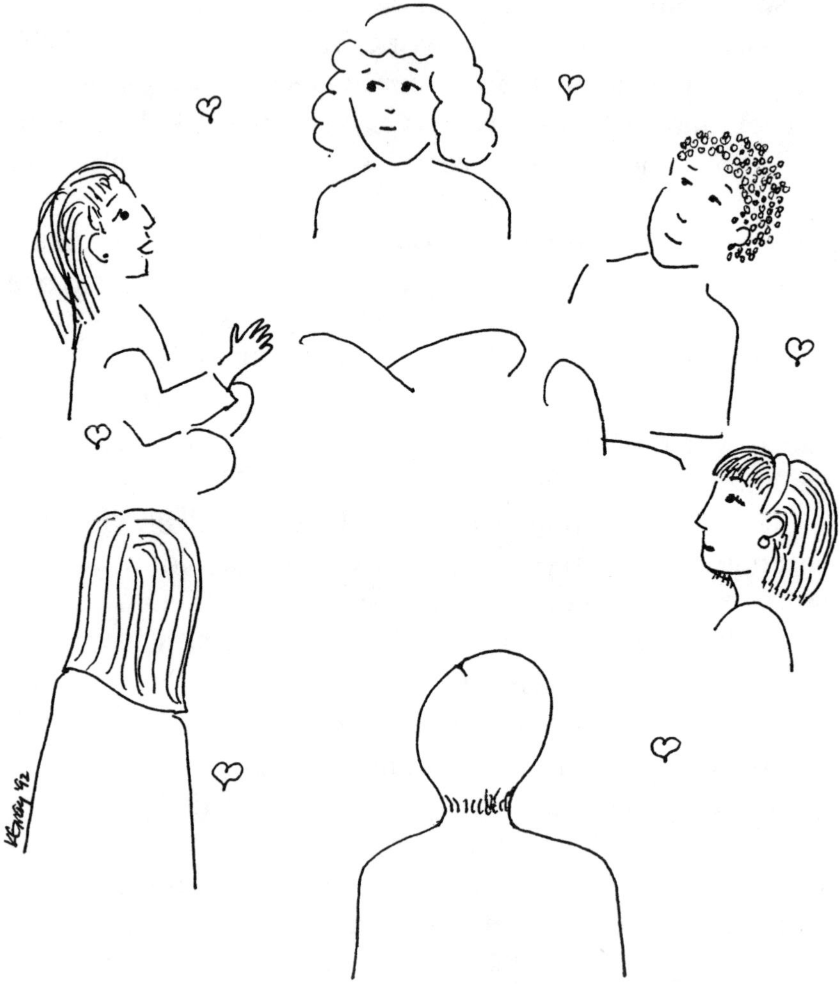

this process works. Of course, the ideal is for the alcoholic/ addict to come to the realization that drinking or using no longer works. Help is indeed as close as the telephone book and volunteers are waiting to talk to the person who finally realizes that life is unmanageable. She must be willing to go to any length to change it. A main vehicle for change is a twelve-step group. If you are already involved in such a group, you are familiar with the steps. Whether or not you are an alcoholic or an addict, the twelve steps are a marvelous way to live. One woman I know who suffers from chronic depression says that the steps have changed her life. She uses them faithfully and as long as she does she feels centered, peaceful and happy. She says, however, "If I stray from the steps, I fall into self-pity and off I go again, into the depression trap." The steps can make all the difference. They are listed and briefly discussed below.

STEP ONE: **We admitted that we were powerless over alcohol, that our lives had become unmanageable.**

Substitute any word you want for the word alcohol. The source of the problem can be many things. It does not have to be simply alcohol. The key word here is POWERLESS. It is only when we are willing to give up our pride, our ego and our old ways of handling things can we begin to "let Go and Let God".

STEP TWO: **Came to believe that a power greater than ourselves could restore us to sanity.**

We do not have to be members of any organized religion. We can be atheists, Christians, Jews, Moslems, or anything else. We need only to admit that we cannot get our lives back in order until we enlist the support of the something or someone greater than ourselves. For many members of the programs, the group itself is the greater than.

STEP THREE: **Made a decision to turn our will and our lives over to the care of God as we understood Him.**

Again, it is the power greater than. Eventually, nearly everyone in the program does find a God of love and acceptance. Often this God is very different than the one we grew up with.

STEP FOUR: **Made a searching and fearless moral inventory of ourselves.**

This step is very hard for most of us, but it is critical. We find, when we are honest about it, that no matter what we had done in the past, we are always acceptable to God. We need only be willing to take the step into self awareness. We find that most of our character defects are the result of fear and anger.

STEP FIVE: **Admitted to God, to ourselves and to another human being the exact nature of our wrongs.**

Oh, how I agonized over this step. I dreaded it. The day I bit the bullet and sat down with my friend Eileen to review my character defects was a most surprising one. I found that she was not shocked by a single thing I told her. She had done or heard it all before. I was relieved of the terrible, heavy load of guilt I had been dragging along behind me for years!

STEP SIX: **Were entirely ready to have God remove all those defects of character.**

Now it is one thing to identify our character defects but another thing entirely to be willing to give them up. We have often become very attached to our habits, unpleasant or unhealthy as they may be. Detach we must, but we don't have to do it alone. We entrust our Higher Power to take them away from us. We only need to be WILLING.

STEP SEVEN: **Humbly ask Him to remove our shortcomings.**

We got down on our knees and prayed. We realized that in order to live life fully and well, we must be ready to let go of the old ways of doing things. We needed to learn what humility is. We had to let go of the old pride which has kept us chained to our addictions. Pride and fear: surely a deadly pair!

STEP EIGHT: **Made a list of all persons we had harmed and became willing to make amends to them all.**

Now we really are on the way to changing the old way of living. We became willing to see where we had been at fault in the troubles we had with family, peers, friends and lovers. We made a commitment to end the isolation of our addiction.

STEP NINE: **Made direct amends to such people wherever possible except when to do so would injure them or others.**

Here we are taking responsibility for our behavior. We need to understand that our lives cannot be free of pain until we have cleared away the wreckage of the past. With this step comes more freedom than can be humanly imagined. A clean conscience is truly a gift of God. In asking forgiveness from others we also come to forgiving ourselves, an essential step on the road to self-love.

STEP TEN: **Continued to take personal inventory and when we were wrong, promptly admitted it.**

We do step ten on a daily basis. This ensures that we never again fall into the trap of self-centeredness which so wrecked our relationships with others in the past. It is not easy to look honestly at our behavior but it can be done and the rewards are great indeed.

STEP ELEVEN: **Sought through prayer and meditation to improve our conscious contact with God as we understood Him, praying only for knowledge of God's will for us and the power to carry that out.**

Self-will is so powerful in us humans. We think we have all the understanding to make good, intellectually sound decisions. And yet, we know so little of the big picture. It is essential that we allow God to direct us. It is not difficult; we only need to pray and trust.

STEP TWELVE: **Having had a spiritual awakening as a result of these steps, we tried to carry this message to others and to practice these principles in all our affairs.**

We go to meetings regularly and by doing so make the message available to anyone who needs to hear it. We speak the truth as we have come to understand it, and and we are willing to share what we have learned with our fellow humans. Most of all, we know that it is only by giving that we receive. By giving our new way of life to others we are ensuring that we keep it for ourselves.

The steps may seem difficult, but they are not. They are the way to live openly, honestly and charitably. We do not have to do the steps alone. We have sponsors who help newcomers do the steps and work the program. It was only when I became willing to commit my life completely to working my program that I came to a sense of peace. Nothing else has ever given me that, though I have searched for answers in many places over many, many years.

From the handout of the Adult Children of Alcoholics, Tucson, Arizona (extracted from writings of Peace Pilgrim), I quote the "Symptoms of Peace" which come from getting involved in a twelve-step program:

"Watch for signs of peace. The hearts of a great many already have been exposed to it and it seems likely that we could find our society experiencing it in epidemic proportions. Some signs and symptoms of inner peace:

1. Tendency to think and act spontaneously rather than from fear.
2. An unmistakable ability to enjoy each moment.
3. Loss of interest in judging other people.
4. Loss of interest in judging self.
5. Loss of interest in interpreting the actions of others.
6. Loss of interest in conflict.
7. Loss of ability to worry.
8. Frequent, overwhelming episodes of appreciation.
9. Contented feelings of connectedness with others and nature.
10. Frequent attacks of smiling through the eyes and from the heart.
11. Interesting tendency to let things happen rather than to make them happen.
12. Increased susceptibility to love extended by others as well as the uncontrollable urge to extend it.

If you have all or even most of the above symptoms, please be advised that your condition may be too far advanced to turn back. If you are exposed at to anyone exhibiting several of these symptoms, remain exposed at your own risk. This Condition of Inner Peace is likely well into its infectious stage. Be forewarned!"

WORKBOOK EXERCISE

End of Chapter Seven.

Answer the following questions with True or False.

1. Most alcoholics/addicts are misfits who cannot hold a job:

2. Alcoholics/addicts rarely achieve financial success in life:

3. It is easy to spot and alcoholic/addict on the job or in a social situation:

4. People who have a problem with alcohol/drugs are weak and losers:

5. Alcoholics/addicts who give up drugs/alcohol are "in recovery":

6. There is no such thing as a "dry drunk":

7. Addiction is limited to alcohol and mood altering chemicals:

8. It is impossible to get an alcoholic/addict to stop drinking or using if he or she is not willing to do so:

9. There is no such thing as addiction to religion or addiction to running:

If you answered "True" to any of the above questions you need to expand your knowledge of addiction and alcoholism.

If you feel you may be in need of recovery work do the following:

1. Get a copy of *Alcoholics Anonymous* (the BIG BOOK) and read it to increase your understanding of the disease of alcohol addiction. The principles discussed can be applied to *any* form of addiction.

2. Call the Central Office of Alcoholics Anonymous and ask to speak to a volunteer about your possible addiction.

3. Make a commitment to your recovery and follow the advice of those who know about the disease. In essence the advice is:

   a) Go to ninety meetings in ninety days.
   b) Get a sponsor.
   c) Work the steps.

Like many wise people who have gone before you, you will get better. Guaranteed!

FURTHER READING

Alcoholics Anonymous: The Story of How Many Men and Women Have Recovered from Alcoholism (AA World Services, Third Edition, 1976). The bible for those who want to learn more about the disease of alcoholism and how to begin their recovery.

Ford, Betty, and Chase, Chris. *Betty: A Glad Awakening.* (Doubleday, 1987). Betty Ford's story of her recovery from alcohol and drug addiction.

Geller, Anne, and Territo, M.J. *Restore Your Life: A Living Plan for Sober People.* (Bantam, 1991). Scholarly, detailed study of alcoholism and recovery.

Olsen, Kristin Gottschalk. *Encyclopedia of Alternative Health Care.* (Pocket Books, 1989). An all-inclusive resource guide that describes many alternative forms of therapy, many of which can be helpful in dealing with addictions.

Self Help Sourcebook: Finding and Forming Mutual Aid Self Help Groups. (Self-Help Clearing House, 1990). This comprehensive national listing of self-help groups also includes a chapter on how you can organize and run a group.

Twelve Steps and Twelve Traditions (AA World Services, 1981). This gem of a work discusses the personal applications of the twelve steps to one's life. A powerful tool for healing.

Chapter 8: I'm O.K.

The Road to Self Love

Discover how beautiful you are, how holy you are. Wherever you walk, there is a blessing that you take with you.

– Tara Singh

I don't precisely know what you need to do to take care of yourself. But I know you can figure it out.

– Melody Beattie

Emotional health is an essential component of high level wellness. It is so easy for us to forget that we too need nurturing and support from ourselves if we are to be happy and well adjusted. We caregivers are so good at giving loving encouragement to the people around us. We are patient, kind and supportive as a matter of routine. That is, when we are caring for others. But to ourselves we often give only intolerant and downright mean messages that negate our self-worth every time we turn around. We do this in every area of our lives and the results can be devastating.

In the many years I have worked as a nurse I have met and worked with a variety of women and men over the country. I don't know how many caregivers I have known, but I would guess that it numbers in the thousands by now. Some I know a lot better than others. The amazing thing to me is that in all those many, many people I can count on one hand the number of them who were really nasty. The reality is that caregivers are decent, good people. The only trouble is that we don't realize our worth.

When we are given unreasonable work loads we may complain about it, but more often we don't. Invariably we do the work to the best of our abilities. It seems to me that rather than congratulating ourselves on having handled a difficult, challenging situation well, we tend to focus on the things we did not get done and beat ourselves up about it. The negative self-messages we give make us feel like failures, and many caregivers simply give up and walk away from their professions because they cannot live up to their own impossibly high performance standards.

Thus, the more we tell ourselves that we are slow, stupid, disorganized or ineffective, the more we will carry these ideas over into our lives. Indeed we create our own experience with our thoughts. Correspondingly, the more positive and uplifting the thoughts, the better reality we will experience. Positive self-messages do wonders for us to handle stress and to perform well on the job.

Pay attention to the way you talk to yourself. When you hear a negative message, STOP! Rephrase the wording of the message to say something positive and uplifting. I assure you, once you start listening, you will be horrified by the kinds of things you habitually say to yourself. They are the statements that you would NEVER use when talking to another human being. So lighten up; love yourself with supportive messages instead of insults.

We seem to get the idea, early in our careers, that we must be all things to all people: we must give all the medications on time; get all the procedures done on time; make all the telephone reports exactly when the doctor wants them; and at the same time we must give full attention to the patients or clients who need our care. I recall going home from a shift in intensive care, feeling so bad because with all the things I had to do for one elderly lady, I just could not find the time to comb her long and tangled hair. When I left work I focused on the one omission and forgot all the positive things I had done for her and two other patients that evening.

It is a health care fact of life that patients need and want the best we can offer. It can be a seemingly simple task, such as brushing their teeth. Despite our good intentions sometimes there just isn't time to perform every possible service. If I continue to beat myself up about what I cannot do, I can easily put myself into a frame of mind which says, "You're a lousy nurse. Get out of this job. You're never good enough. Let someone else worry about it."

Where does this anxiety come from? Lots of sources. One is the nurse educator. Many of the nursing instructors I have known have established impossibly high standards of performance for students. The irony is that most of these same instructors had abandoned bedside nursing themselves. Many have told me that the job of the staff nurse "was just too tough." Hence, they moved out of the hospital environment and into academia. These often disenchanted staff nurses are in a position of authority over students. They say what *must* be done by the aspiring professional. Frequently their requirements are excessive with no room allowed for the difficulty of meeting those requirements as a matter of daily clinical routine. In my view, it would be ideal if nurse educators spent several weeks each year actually applying the standards that they teach by working as staff nurses. This would provide two main benefits for the profession. First, the educators would learn first-hand the role of today's staff nurse. Second, the infusion of more nurses into the system on a regular basis would bring more badly-needed staff into situations where many nurses are overworked on a daily basis.

When they are students, young nurses function in an environment which supports thoroughness of care. They are able to do everything that should be done for their patients while they are in nursing school. They have only one or two patients each. They not only have their nursing instructor close at hand but also an RN mentor who is responsible for that patient. I have seen their shock and despair when they first begin as staff nurses and find out that they simply *cannot do* all the things that they were taught were essential. They now have many patients, some very sick, who require much care. How is it possible to give everything to everyone? It simply is not.

The first year on the job is critical and many eager young caregivers burn out because they never learn to forgive themselves for being human. They have to cut corners. They have to prioritize, do what must be done and leave the rest. No one can be the perfect nurse who knows everything and does everything which should be done on every shift. We must learn to set reasonable standards for ourselves. It seems an extremely difficult thing to do, but the simple fact is that our jobs require that we do our best. That's all. WE are the ones who tell ourselves that we cannot under any circumstances, make any mistakes or do less than what we would like during a shift.

Perhaps other professional caregivers "drop out" of their jobs as fast as hospital staff nurses do but I doubt it. We are so hard on ourselves, and the job can be so physically and emotionally exhausting, that we leave at alarming rates.

We must love ourselves enough to allow for being human. No, we are not perfect. We are committed to caring for others; let us commit to caring for ourselves too. It is also important for us to give loving support to our colleagues. I have seen vast differences in the way that various nursing units work together. The most demanding workloads with the most difficult patients are bearable when staff care about one another and show that they do. It is particularly important to encourage new graduates as they struggle with their difficult transition. We need to make a point of noticing what new people on the job do well and tell them so. Notice people doing things right and reward them with positive strokes.

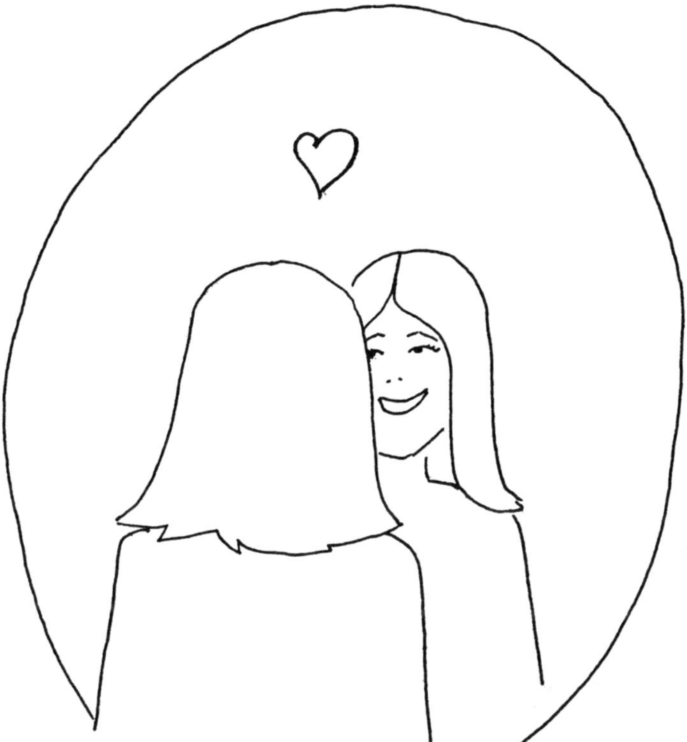

Chances are they will repeat the behavior time and time again. Of course the reverse is true. Put simply, negativity will beget negativity.

But remember, you are important. *You* must accept that you are doing the best you possibly can and that it is okay. By serving others in your work, you are blessing everyone whose lives you touch. Loving yourself and accepting your humanity is essential, if you are to function successfully in this world.

WORKBOOK EXERCISE

End of Chapter Eight

Answer the following questions with "Yes" or "No":

1. I always speak kindly to myself:

2. When I make a mistake I admit it honestly, rectify it and forgive myself for being human:

3. I smile at myself whenever I look in the mirror:

4. Never do I call myself names like Stupid and Dummy:

5. I always congratulate myself on a job well done:

6. When someone gives me a compliment of any kind, I am gracious about receiving it:

7. It is easy for me to receive public praise:

8. When my boss finds fault with my work or my behavior on the job, and I know she is correct, I accept her input and strive to improve my performance:

9. I can say with all sincerity that I LOVE MYSELF and that I am okay:

10. It is easy for me to nurture and care for myself in body, mind and spirit.

If you have answered "No" to any of the above questions you may want to work on improving your self-talk and the way you view yourself.

1. Pay attention to the way you talk to yourself in your mind. If you notice any negative messages to YOU, stop immediately and rephrase them to be loving, nurturing and supportive. As you do this more and more consistently you will feel better about yourself no matter what is going on in your life.

2. Every day spend two minutes looking directly into your own face in the mirror. As you look into the image, tell that person that you love and support her, always. Hold the eye contact. Look lovingly at yourself. Then give yourself a big hug with both arms.

Doesn't that feel good? Love yourself a lot; you deserve it!

FURTHER READING

Bolen, Jean Shinoda. *Goddesses in Every Woman.* (Harper, 1985). Discusses archetypes of women, using Greek goddesses as models. Based on the ideas of Carl Jung.

Chopra, Deepak. *Quantum Healing: Exploring the Frontiers of Mind/Body Healing.* (Bantam, 1989). Fascinating book synthesizes current developments in Western medicine, neuroscience, Ayurveda (Indian medicine), and quantum physics.

Cohen, Alan. *Dare to be Yourself.* (Alan Cohen Publications, 1990). A book on finding your inner strength and empowering yourself to live more fully in the present.

Jampolsky, Gerald. *Love is Letting Go of Fear* (Celestial Arts, 1979). A small but powerful book which can change your self-talk.

Maltz, Maxwell. *Psycho-Cybernetics* (Prentice-Hall, 1960). A tried and true volume for improving your personal power.

Murphy, Joseph. *The Power of Your Subconscious Mind* (Bantam, 1982). Identifies words and phrases which are negative and shows us how to change them.

Chapter 9: Speaking Up

Assertiveness and Emotional Health

Each of us has the ability to make the world a better place.

– Claudia Black

Assertion is a skill to be learned, not a quality we're born with like long legs.

– Sonya Friedman

One way for caregivers to maintain and increase a good, healthy level of emotional wellness is by learning assertiveness skills. Some caregivers seem to possess a natural ability to speak up for themselves and for their patients, but unfortunately, many of us burn out because we lack the ability to do so.

I've observed that a common behavior among caregivers is the passive-aggressive mode of dealing with life. We tend to tolerate uncomfortable situations and unreasonable demands long past the time when we might have spoken up. Then, all of a sudden, there is an outburst of anger and frustration. It happens with staffing schedules, with workloads and assignments, all manner of things. Even though we have learned what assertiveness is, we often lack the ability or determination to practice it.

Obviously, we all perceive reality differently, but the basic reality of assertiveness is speaking one's own truth. Others have no way of knowing just what is going on for us unless we have the courtesy of sharing that with them. We need to use what is often termed "I messages." Without attacking her, we can tell the boss how we feel about our situation. "I feel upset because I have been scheduled to work three weekends in a row." On the other hand, attacking a supervisor in the middle of a busy work area or when she is occupied in a meeting is inappropriate. It will not endear one to her, no matter how good a clinician the staff member is.

Being assertive means identifying your feelings, before they get out of control, and sharing them with the appropriate person in the proper place and at the proper time. Keeping your complaints to yourself is defeating in the extreme. I have often quoted my dear departed grandmother with her statement, "The squeaky wheel gets the grease." Put another way, if you don't squeak, you'll never get the grease, i.e. what you want.

One way staff members exhibit passive-aggressive behavior is when they complain to everyone except the right person. Not only do they rule out the possibility of getting what they want, but they cause a real morale problem in the workplace. It is not necessary to put anyone else down in order to be assertive. That is why the "I messages" are important. In this way no one can be defensive as no one is being attacked. The other person is free to respond without the need to defend herself . No unnecessary conflict results from this honest, open type of communication.

Assertiveness has not been the easiest thing in the world for me to learn and I don't think I am unlike a lot of other caregivers. In my case, I grew up with the admonition that children are to be seen but not heard. I was taught to respect my elders and anyone else who had authority over me. Being a "good girl" meant being submissive and overly agreeable to everyone, often at the cost of my needs. I rarely expressed anger and was very much afraid of conflict. If I was unhappy with a situation I would complain about it indirectly and if things were not resolved, I became resentful and depressed. As I grew older, the basic process repeated itself in my work life and personal life. I've learned that wherever we are, we need to express our requests and needs directly or they will never be met.

Rokelle Lerner writes that anger unexpressed kills love, kills passion and kills relationships. I really believe that is true. Holding resentment inside kills us, little by little. Our only hope is to learn to speak our truth with courage. Somehow, I think caregivers find it easier to speak up for our clients and patients. My role as patient advocate has been one of the most satisfying parts of my nursing career. Again, it is not an easy thing for us to face conflict, but when we do it for a helpless patient we can summon reserves of courage we did not know we had. When we go out on a limb and speak assertively it seems well worth the risk.

So many patients come into hospitals with no idea at all of their rights as health care consumers. The American Hospital Association has prepared a "Patient Bill of Rights" which is available in any accredited hospital. Unfortunately, most patients aren't even aware that this document exists. It says that the patient is the one who should be in control of his care. He ALWAYS has the right to say "NO". Younger patients often know that, but most of the elderly do not.

I remember one sweet little elderly female patient who once asked me in wonderment about a conversation she had just overheard in the intensive care unit where she was a patient. A young man, dying of alcohol induced pancreatitis, had loudly refused to have a nasogastric tube placed through his nose into his stomach. He was very distended and obviously needed the tube to relieve the pressure in his gut. But he had been in the hospital many times and he knew his rights. He would not agree to the procedure. He subsequently died and probably would have whether or not the tube was in place. The lady said to me, "Can we do that? Can we really say no to something the doctor wants to do to us?"

It was my pleasure to inform her of her rights as a

consumer. She is an autonomous individual who has ultimate responsibility for her body. She can say NO to anything that does not seem right to her. She does need to know the ramifications of her decisions and needs to be mentally competent. A loving, supportive family who agrees to her wishes is a great benefit; with support she will be empowered to get what she wants from the medical system, and refuse what she does not want.

We nurses need to be supportive of other members of the health care team, but not when it clearly violates the wishes of the patient. It takes time to develop the skills necessary to act as a patient advocate, but I have seen even relatively inexperienced nurses act very decisively and courageously in helping the patient who is up against the combined powers of the system. Fortunately, today's caregivers are well educated and prepared to confront the care providers - be they individuals or institutions - who fail to respect the rights of the individual and the family.

Historically, nurses have consistently taken a stand for patient rights in the areas of hospital visitation rules, patient education, childbirth preparation, family-centered maternity, hospice care and many others. We can be assertive, diligent and very successful in speaking up for patients. We must be every bit as consistent in speaking up for ourselves.

Yes, it is necessary to talk about doctors at this point. We seem to have an inordinate amount of difficulty in dealing with those folks. I am happy to say that doctors are a lot easier to work with today than they were when I came into the field in the fifties. Believe it or not, back then we had to stand up when a doctor entered the nurses' station. If we were busy in the middle of charting, no matter. Stop what you are doing and pay respects (the analogy to officers and the military is instructive). We were taught to stand aside and let the MD's go first into the elevator. We had never even heard the term "assertiveness", much less tried it on a physician. We were taught simply to be hand-maidens.

At the same time, the patient was not allowed to know anything at all about his condition or his care, unless he heard it from The Doctor. When we took vital signs we were forbidden to tell the patient what his temperature, pulse or blood pressure was. The standard reply was "you'll have to talk to your doctor." The same was true of any medications we gave. We might have said, "it is for your blood pressure," but we were never to divulge the name of the drug or the dosage. Certainly the side effects always remained a mystery to the patient unless the doctor took the time to tell him.

Things have changed; the doctor is no longer the sole and ultimate authority in matters of health care. Yes, he has his area of expertise, but the plain truth is that there is so vast a pool of medical knowledge today that no one person can possibly master and dispense all of it. The physician must enlist the expertise of many disciplines in order to meet the needs of his patients. He must call upon the skills of the pharmacist, physical therapist, occupational therapist, speech therapist, social worker and the nurse, in addition to many others. All caregivers have a powerful voice on the team today and that does my heart good, as we have so much to share. If the doctor wants the best for his patient and really takes responsibility for that, he cheerfully enlists the support of the entire health care team.

Today doctors are still primarily trained as scientists. They understand the complex chemistry, anatomy and physiology of the human body. Nurses, on the other hand, with far less purely scientific training, are eminently capable of handling complex patient assessment, intervention and evaluation. The doctors' discovery of this fact has caused them to better appreciate the nurse as a full team member. And while they may not always show enough respect for the ability of the general staff nurse, they have come a long, long way. They are much more approachable. The assertive nurse, when she speaks from her education and experience, is usually heard by today's physician.

It is not to say that this is consistently the case. I have experienced the kind of abuse and harassment which has driven many promising nurses out of the field. There are times when the behavior of the doctor ranges from insensitive and unprofessional to downright insane in the way he treats his fellow caregivers. This does not make sense at all, given the fact that without the nursing staff (and of course the other staff as well) he cannot possibly take care of his patients.

Hospital administration has a duty to support, with equal respect, all the professionals who practice within the institution. Unfortunately, it is a fact of life that the physician is the one who controls the patient entry into the system. He is the one who determines the actual census of the hospital. Naturally, the MD who consistently provides the institution with the greatest number of patients is the one who gets the most respect by the folks who run the place. It becomes a real ethical dilemma when the most "productive" doctor begins to cause serious morale problems by his aggressive behavior towards hospital staff.

I remember very well a plastic surgeon who wielded his power like a well-sharpened sword around the hospital where I had taken a position as a head nurse. He was pampered by the hospital administration and could get away with absolutely outrageous behavior simply because he was good at what he did. He admitted his patients to our hospital exclusively and he made a lot of money for the institution. The unit where his patients were admitted was a mixture of pediatrics and medical/surgical adults. There were so many problems on the unit that there was no one in the hospital who was willing to take the head nurse position when it became available.

Without realizing what I was getting into, I interviewed and got the job. I recall that one of the questions I was asked

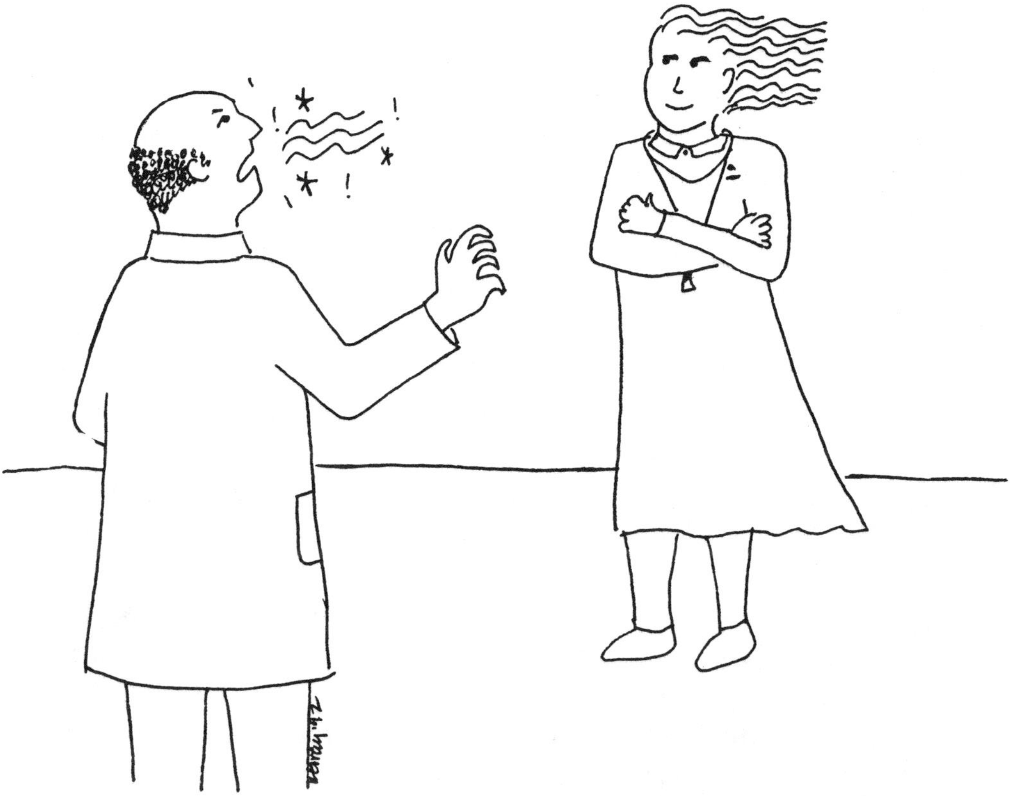

referred to this particular doctor and what his reputation meant to me. I had no negative notions about him and had found him to be a competent surgeon and a man of personal integrity. The first time I experienced this man's foul temper I was astonished. He came totally unglued over a minor lapse in admission protocol and subsequently became a roaring bull elephant (he was a large fellow), tearing a wide swath from my unit all the way to the administration. He charged us all with being stupid, among other unflattering things, and left for the operating room after his impressive scene.

When he came back to the unit later he was in fine spirits. It was as though nothing had happened at all. Everyone on the floor was tense and anxious, wondering what would happen next. As we walked together into the hallway, I confronted him. I was quiet but firm.

I said, "I really don't appreciate being called stupid. I was upset that you caused such a scene this morning."

He looked surprised and his neck began to flush. He replied: "I didn't call you stupid."

"No," I replied, "not specifically. But you said everyone here was stupid and that naturally includes me."

He did not apologize but he did say magnanimously, "Well, I think you're going to be the perfect head nurse for this unit!"

My answer to that comment was simply: "No, I will never be perfect. No one is. But I will do the best possible job for our patients and so will my staff."

The interesting thing is that man never did pull a stunt like that again in the two years I was head nurse on the unit. He fussed and even shouted occasionally but never caused such a ruckus again. Perhaps he had been testing the new head nurse. Whatever his purpose, we got to understand one another. He was and probably still is a big bully. Any time we give in without asserting ourselves with people like that, we are doomed to more and/or worse treatment in the future.

Bullies don't respect the folks they can push around.

One of the things that all of us need to remember is that doctors are just people. They have the same human needs for recognition, love, acceptance and respect that the rest of us do. Granted, some of them seem to demand more than their share of the above, using some bizarre ways to achieve it. But basically they're vulnerable, just as we are. They want to be heard and they want their patients to do well. They get frustrated when things don't go the way they want. They get tired, grumpy, difficult and demanding. Theirs is not an easy road, though it sometimes looks that way to others. A little kindness, support and understanding will go a long way in making for a happy working relationship between physicians and the rest of the health care team.

It is important to speak the truth, as you see it, to any care provider with whom you work. It does not mean that you must hit anyone over the head with it. Showing tolerance and consideration is never out of line. It is unfair to sabotage a doctor's efforts simply out of fear of confronting him directly. Better to be open, honest and loving. Everyone can win when everyone plays fair. Most of all, the health care consumer deserves the very best that we can give him by working together and supporting one another for the good of our patients and clients.

WORKBOOK EXERCISE

End of Chapter Nine

Answer the following questions with a "Yes" or "No":

1. I am very clear about the meaning of the word as*sertive*:

2. I know the difference between assertive and aggressive:

3. I am always assertive in making my needs known:

4. I never use manipulation in my dealings with others:

5. If I have a complaint about anything at work I take it to the appropriate person:

6. I speak directly to the person with whom I have an issue and no one else:

7. It is easy for me to disagree with someone if I need to do so:

8. If someone tries to engage me in a conversation which is negative or unkind, I promptly change the subject or tell the person I choose not to discuss it:

9. Outside of my work place I speak well of my colleagues and the institution for which I work, or I do not speak of them:

10. If I am concerned about the behavior of a peer or a physician I always confront the person honestly and directly:

If you answered "No" to two or more of the questions above, you may wish to work on improving your assertiveness skills.

Choose one of the following books and read it:

Alberti, Robert E., and Emmons, Michael. *Your Perfect Right: A Guide to Assertive Living*. (Impact Publishers, 1986).

Dyer, Wayne. *Pulling Your Own Strings.* (Harper Perennial, 1991).

Friedman, Sonya. *Smart Cookies Don't Crumble: A Woman's Guide to Living and Loving Her Own Life.* (Putnam, 1985).

Lloyd, Sam. *Developing Positive Assertiveness.* (Crisp Publications, 1988).

McFarland, Rhoda. *Coping Through Assertiveness.* (Rosen Publishing Group, 1986).

Practice being assertive in small, easy situations like complaining about food you don't like in a restaurant. As you develop skill in easy areas you can do the more difficult ones like confronting an authority figure or an aggressive person.

Chapter 10: Producer, Director and Star

Creating Your Own Experience

We have our brush and colors - paint paradise and in we go.

– Nikos Kazantzakis

Most people are about as happy as they make up their minds to be.

– Abraham Lincoln

It is a funny thing about life; if you refuse to accept anything but the best, you very often get it.

– Somerset Maugham

The emotionally healthy person has a life which is well balanced, satisfying and serene. No matter what kind of events are taking place all around her, she views the world in a way which promotes positivity rather than negativity. Happiness comes from "an attitude of gratitude," as they say in twelve-step programs. We each see reality in a different way; no two people view things exactly the same. Our genetics, our history and our personal way of dealing with life is highly individualized.

I believe that life as each one of us sees it is merely a projection of what is going on inside the individual. If we want to change what is going on in our lives, we cannot focus around the "screen" (the outer world) and make any meaningful changes. It is essential that we work on the "projector" (our way of looking at things) in order to make a real impact. By simply changing the way we look at life we change our experience of it. That is why we can surely say that our thoughts create our reality. Think negative thoughts often enough and we create a negative experience.

Inasmuch as we caregivers are under a lot of stress as we go about our daily chores, research has shown that it is not the stress itself which causes serious problems for the people who are in the middle of it. The problems come from our PERCEPTION OF THE STRESS. In other words, it is not the situation which is making us sick or fatigued, it is the way we view ourselves within the situation and the emotion we attach to what is going on.

Caregivers vary greatly in the way each of us views the world. Our view is affected by our state of health, energy and our mood. I know that when I arrive at work well rested, with no big pressures ongoing on at home, I have a fairly rosy view of how I'm going to handle my shift. Regardless of what they tell me in the report, I believe that I can handle the situation and I usually do. But if I arrive at work tired, feeling low, or with something on my mind, I see a monster lurking in every corner. I view reality as being very threatening and anxiety-producing. I fear all the scary possibilities (whether or not I show it to others) and usually end up creating problems for myself simply because of my fearful attitude.

I have experimented with positive thinking on the way to work and it really makes a difference in the way things go. I say some affirmations as I walk along like, "Today I am going to have a productive, happy shift. Things will go well for me today. I am a well organized nurse; today will be a good day." And you know, it usually works out just that way.

It is not just my experience which tells me that a positive attitude works. I have shared my ideas with other caregivers and they too have found that by focusing on the positive possibilities, they tend to experience more of them. If they worry about having "codes" or conflicts, they usually have them. Controlling the way we think is critical if we want to have a satisfying and rewarding time at work.

In every aspect of our lives we can find ourselves feeling more balanced, secure and content simply by paying attention to what we are thinking. We can use the time when we are waiting in line at the super market to relax, do some deep breathing and think uplifting thoughts.

We can send happy thoughts to the people around us and far away as well. We do not have to poison our reality with negatives like, "Boy, this line is so slow today. I'm going to be so late getting home. Supper will be so bad because I don't have time to prepare a decent meal. I can't stand to waste time like this. What is the matter with that clerk anyway? She must be new on the job; she can't seem to get it together."

Of course our thoughts don't remain where they are in our minds. They take flight and become real objects which have power to wreak havoc on the people around us. By sending peaceful, loving thoughts to the same clerk, you will empower her to perform her job better and you will make yourself feel good at the same time. Your emotional health can be improved immeasurably simply by watching what you think.

Gratitude is probably the most powerful emotion I know to transform one's attitude. When I am feeling unhappy about my life I can change everything in just a few minutes. I take out my pencil and paper and begin a gratitude list. I write down everything that comes into my mind. It usually looks something like this:

I am grateful for:
the bright sunny day
the soft breezes
the tall, green trees swaying in the wind
the sounds of life all around me, birds, children, people
the smell of the fresh air
the brightly colored flowers

my healthy, strong body
my good mind
my wonderful children (I name each one)
my supportive, loving family, especially my sisters (I name each one)
my dear kind special friends (I name every one I can think of)
my beloved husband
and on and on!

The page fills up fast! How can I possibly feel miserable with a list like that!? I have absolutely nothing to feel sorry for myself anymore.

Believe it or not, it is even possible to do that in the work situation. When I am feeling swamped or somewhat angry about how things are going on the job, a gratitude list makes all the difference. I may have to write the list while I am eating my sandwich at lunch or at home after I have finished work, but it always gets me on the right track. The gratitude list looks something like this:

my strong legs for running all shift long
my healthy body for being capable of hard work
my fine mind for being able to solve clinical problems
my supportive peers for helping me get finished my work
our unit secretary for staying cool in the midst of chaos
the family who stayed with a patient and helped with her care
the pharmacy for getting my orders out so fast
the lab for getting the blood ready when I needed it
the doctor who got what he needed unassisted
my supervisor for her supportive concern
and on and on.

Suddenly my attitude is transformed not because things happened differently, but because I have changed the way I looked at what happened. Truly amazing! I am encouraged to go on and learn from my experience. If I get stuck in negativity, I find myself in a very bad place. I see only the bad,

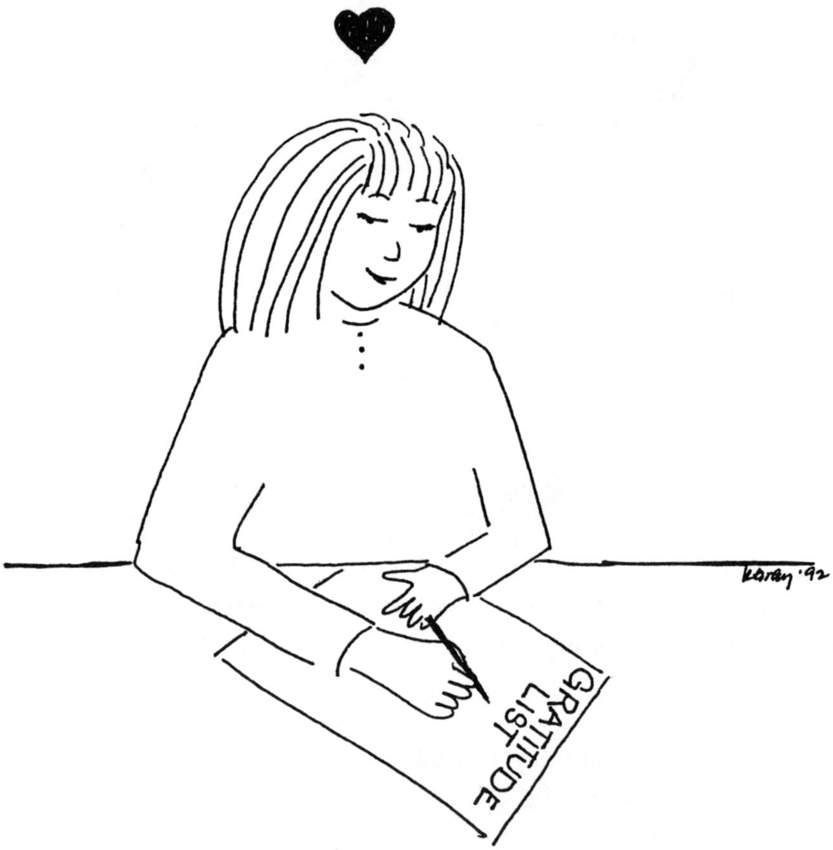
GRATITUDE LIST

the depressing, the difficult. But life isn't like that. No matter how hard things are, there is always something to be grateful for.

The best story I have ever heard about gratitude comes from the book, The *Hiding Place*, by Corrie ten Boom with John and Elizabeth Sherrill. In the book Corrie recounts her experience in Ravensbruck concentration camp during World War II. She and her saintly sister Betsy had been imprisoned in that dreadful place for having helped Dutch Jews escape the Nazis. Each evening, after a long, miserable day at forced labor, the sisters led a prayer group and bible study in the midst of the filth and horror of the camp. They always closed the evening with a list of things for which they were thankful during the day. One night Corrie was shocked to hear her sister say, "And thank you God for the fleas." Corrie could not restrain her indignation and chastised Betsy for such a remark. But Betsy replied, "But Corrie, in the Bible it says we must give thinks for ALL things." Corrie grumbled and accepted the explanation. Much to her amazement, they later learned that the only reason the vicious guards did not come into their bunk areas to harass and beat them was because they were afraid of the fleas!

Attitude changes everything. We all know people who have managed to grow and blossom and keep peaceful despite formidable challenges in their lives. And then there are others who have nothing good, uplifting or positive to say about anything. I talked with a social worker recently who is looking for a part-time job to supplement her retirement income. She is bright, capable and talented. As we spoke about the various job possibilities which are available to her I realized that she will never find a job which pleases her. She does not believe that it is possible. No matter what we discussed, she could only see the negative in the job. Never did she focus on a positive idea. She is creating a reality and it will not be a pleasant one. That is her choice.

The truth is that no matter what goes on in our lives we choose how we will react. Two different people look at the same glass of water and each one sees something different, depending on her attitude. One sees a glass half empty, the other sees a glass half full. It is only a point of view, but it makes all the difference.

One way for us to learn to view our work challenges as opportunities rather than threats is to select professional role models and mentors. In every place where I have worked there has been at least one caregiver who had an unfailingly positive attitude. Sometimes there are many. What is it that makes them so cheerful in the midst of what seems like great stress? How can they manage to juggle all the demands being placed on them and yet have time to provide a helping hand to the younger, less experienced professionals? Often, their strength lies in their clinical expertise, but that alone does not make them special. What truly makes the difference is that these people have a positive attitude. They focus on what is good about the work rather than the problems. They honor the skills of their peers; rarely do they waste time and energy complaining about problems.

I will never forget Sister Maria Goretti, who was head nurse on a very busy pediatric unit where I worked, soon after my graduation. She was not much older than me but she had much more clinical expertise. That was not what made her special, though. It was her amazing optimism in the face of almost impossible odds. We were faced with very similar problems which are still present in acute care facilities: shortage of well qualified staff, demanding physicians, heavy work loads, and high staff turnover with an often crushing load of sick patients. And we did not have intensive care units then.

It did not matter what kind of situation this woman faced, she could always find something good to say about it. It was not that she was a Pollyanna. She was very feisty and could stand up to any kind of pressure from whatever direction it came. We had a patient load which consisted of kids from a few days old to late teens. Sometimes we even took adults because of bed shortages on adult units. One day I was shocked to learn that Admitting wanted to place not one but two critically ill adults in iron lungs on our unit.

Iron lungs had originally been developed for the care of polio patients who could not breathe on their own. The devices were rarely used after polio had largely been eradicated by the Salk vaccine. Ventilators were just coming into use at that time and for some reason, none were available in the hospital. Because of the special needs of those two patients, two old iron lungs were resurrected from the hospital cellar and put into use. No one on our unit had ever cared for a critically ill patient totally sheathed in a huge metal cocoon before.

We were all aghast. Of course they did not plan to give us any more staff in order to care for these additional patients. We wondered what Sister would say about it. But her response was quick in coming. She looked a bit surprised for a moment, but then she said, "Oh good. Now we will get to learn all about taking care of patients in iron lungs."

Nothing fazed her. She was always ready to lend a helping hand and could be depended upon as a source of encouragement and virtually unending patience. She was my mentor and role model for the years I worked with her. Under her firm but gentle guidance I learned more about being a good nurse than I thought possible. Never did she put me down. I grew to be calm, confident and capable, and her many good lessons have remained with me for the more than a quarter century since we worked together.

Everywhere, there are these special people in the health care field, willing to share and to lead. Look around and you will see them. Often they are modest and don't realize how inspiring they are. They are not necessarily the head nurses on the units, though sometimes this is the case. I have worked with some multi-talented and helpful licensed practical nurses and nursing assistants who have taught me much about nursing. It is not that they set out to do that. But through their competence and dedication, they role model professionalism at its best.

Focus on these leaders, learn from them and you will find yourself feeling better about yourself and your job. When you feel secure and peaceful inside, everything goes better. There is a sense of security which is the inevitable product of this kind of growth. As they say, imitation is the sincerest form of flattery. To this I would add that imitation in the best sense can go a long way in the areas of self-maintenance and general wellness.

No matter what we do to take care of our emotional well being to feel happier on the job and in our personal life, there is one more thing that must be said. That is, REMAIN IN THE MOMENT. Stay there both at work and at home and you will avoid many unnecessary moments of pain. Of course we all have to plan our work and our lives to some extent, but once the outline is complete, let go of it. Focus on the now; notice everything about what is going on at this particular moment. That is, really EXPERIENCE the moment. I have found that when I do that, wherever I am, I live more fully and happily than I ever imagined. If I focus on the past, I can get very quickly into guilt and regret. If I move into the future, fear and anxiety await me. But if I stay in the moment, everything is fine. Only in this sense can we create our own experience, as experience can only exist in the *now*, and never in the past or the future.

So take time to appreciate yourself and what you are doing to contribute to the betterment of our world. No matter where we are or what we do, we do make a difference. We all matter greatly in the scheme of things, so let's give ourselves a pat on the back. Self-appreciation works wonders.

WORKBOOK EXERCISE

End of Chapter Ten

Answer the following questions with a "Yes" or "No":

1. I have a very optimistic attitude about life:

2. Every job I have ever had has been an enriching experience:

3. I can always see the gift in any problem which is presented in life:

4. I am grateful for the way my life is right now:

5. Even though I work very hard, I am satisfied with my job and my professional life in general:

6. Each day I notice the good things in my life and I give thanks for them:

7. I feel serene and peaceful no matter what is going on around me:

8. I have worked with several individuals who have inspired me with their positive attitudes:

9. I make a difference for people and I am glad about that:

10. I have been told that my attitude and behavior role model a high standard of professionalism:

If you answered "No" to two or more of the above questions, please do the following exercises:

1. When you are feeling stressed out or unhappy in area of your life, sit down and write out a gratitude list as soon as you can find time. It will change your attitude immediately.

2. Begin to notice the good things happening around you. Say "Thanks" to the people you work with and compliment them when you see them doing something well. It must be sincere, otherwise don't bother. People recognize flattery eventually.

3. Write a note of appreciation to someone who has inspired you. Just a few words of thanks will make you feel good and will be a great blessing to the person who receives it. Do this at least once a month, more often if appropriate.

4. If you are a manager, make a point to recognize the contribution of your employees on a regular basis. You will be glad you did.

FURTHER READING

Allenbaugh, Eric. *Wake Up Calls.* (Discovery Publications, 1991). Recognizing challenges as opportunity and growing in the process.

Delaney, Gayle. *Living Your Dreams.* (Harper & Row, 1988). Simply written book which helps us to use dreams to solve problems and enrich our lives.

King, Laurel. *Women of Power.* (Celestial Arts, 1989). Profiles ten women associated with metaphysical and spiritual teachings. Among those discussed are Louise Hay, Elisabeth Kubler-Ross and Lynn Andrews.

Ornstein, Robert and Sobel, David. *Healthy Pleasures* (Addison-Wesley, 1989). Examines the role of pleasure in health and general well being. Refreshingly written in a lively, jargon-free style, the book delivers the common sense message that health flows naturally from within when we practice the things which bring us joy.

Williamson, Marianne. *A Return to Love.* (Harper, 1992). Sheds light on the principles of *A Course in Miracles* and how to use them. An excellent and inspiring book.

Chapter 11: Friends and Lovers

Relationships and Other Challenges

True self-love is the foundation of all other relationships.

– St. Germaine

Communicate clearly with love, honesty, truth, a willingness to be seen and with compassion and wisdom to the best of your capacity.

– Emmanuel

We first learn about relationships in our family of origin. Unfortunately, when the family is dysfunctional, we do not learn healthy, honest, open ways of communicating with one another. We learn a lot about manipulation, control, fear and people pleasing. Developing a healthy, intimate, equal relationship later in life is difficult when we start out without the right kind of information.

Whether parents teach by word or example, there is constant teaching and constant learning. We learn many different ways of dealing with the world. These behaviors become a part of our "tool kit" for dealing with life as we go along. Many of them are very useful ways of coping but some are not. There comes a time when we are forced to look at what we've learned. We need to decide which behaviors belong in the kit and which ones must be discarded. I learned many good things from my parents. I was taught how to be dependable, hard-working, neat and loyal, but I also learned some unhealthy behaviors.

From my mother I learned that men were very useful but that one had to be constantly on guard lest they somehow get the upper hand and take advantage. I learned that I must choose an appropriate spouse who would take care of me. Through him I was to get all of my needs met. It would be okay to choose a diamond in the rough, just as long as I realized that it would be a lifetime commitment to mold him into the kind of husband who could make me proud. A man was to provide me with a beautiful home, children, clothing and a position in the community. She also made it clear that it would be a good idea for me to have a good education "just in case" I ever needed to work, as it would be helpful to have a marketable skill. Mother was right about a lot of things. Considering her old school generation, she had a good understanding of how things worked in those days.

She taught me to guard my body against male intrusion upon it. They want one thing, she would say, and after that they are no longer interested in you. She said that it was a good thing to go out with a lot of different boys so that I would learn what it was I wanted in a spouse. So I did. I never allowed anyone to get too close to me, to get to know the real person inside. I maintained a facade of ladylike perfection combined with sensual desirability. This protected me from total involvement with any man, ever.

Because I practiced what I was taught, I managed to have twenty-five years of marriage without ever really developing true adult intimacy. I stifled all of my feelings and became so good at doing that, I did not even know what I felt. Anger was buried deep inside of me; it became depression. I learned that if you wanted to get something from a man, you must never be direct. You must use subtle manipulation and feigned helplessness. Make him think it is his idea. It worked. I married a man who was vulnerable to my kind of behavior and through him I achieved every goal I wanted, at great personal cost to both of us. Only much later in life did I learn that the only way to have a real, live relationship is to share what is going on inside, and to express needs, feelings and even resentments honestly, openly, and in a mutually supportive atmosphere of love and caring.

From my father I learned that I was never good enough because I was female. He taught me many good things: how to speak properly; how to take my education seriously; and how to strive to be the best I could at everything I did. If I brought home a report card with four A's and one B, the B got all the attention. But he also taught me other things. Prominent among them was how to fear: men, authority and my feelings. He believed that to "spare the rod meant to spoil the child." He took his role as a parent very seriously. We were not "spoiled."

I realize now that when I came into this lifetime, I chose those particular parents in order to learn the lessons I needed to master. But for years I felt a lot of anger because of my painful childhood. I could hardly wait to get out of my home and be on my own. Now I know it was perfect for my learning and I can thank both my parents for providing an ideal environment for growth. I realize that my parents did much better than theirs had done for them. Both of them had come from dysfunctional, abusive families. No one taught them how to parent and they had no healthy role models to follow.

My parents were unhappy, frustrated people. They never learned how to love and nurture themselves or each other. They were not able to get what they needed in their relationship. How could they possibly provide children with the unconditional love and support which is the right of every child who comes into this world? For them happiness was so elusive. They did not learn how to create it for themselves much less for their children. They did not know they deserved to be happy.

Today, we are fortunate to have so much more information available to us. Bookstores overflow with volumes and volumes of writings on the family and relationships. There are classes, support groups and virtually endless opportunities to learn how to do better in all our parenting and relating to other humans. Things are improving as more and more of us learn how to love one another better. To paraphrase St. Germaine, to have a good relationship with anyone else, we must first have a good one with ourselves.

In years past, young adults married, raised families and remained together "until death us do part". Today, it is tempting to see divorce statistics as proof that we don't know how to have solid relationships anymore. But I am not so sure. I recall being horrified, back in the 1960s, when I read an article written by anthropologist Margaret Mead. She said that people ought to plan for serial marriages rather than for one long relationship. Her reasoning was: because of the increased longevity of North Americans, it is very unlikely that two people would or could maintain a mutually satisfying marriage over the long lifetimes we now enjoy. It appears that Margaret knew what she was talking about. Although the divorce rate remains high, so does the rate of remarriage. No matter what we may think about marriage as an institution, statistics and studies suggest that people have better health and longer lives in marriages rather than outside them.

Today, I believe that "till death us do part" might be interpreted as the death of the marriage rather than the death of the spouse. Once the union becomes uncomfortable and lacks the nurturing support which it much have for both partners, something needs to be done about it. Counseling is often helpful, but if one partner has psychologically or physically abandoned the relationship there is rarely any point in trying to make it work.

The primary purpose for a relationship is to serve as an opportunity for growth for both partners. Despite all appearances, I believe that we choose partners who will help us master lessons. Our partners serve as mirrors; we choose exactly the kind of people we need in order to learn and grow. If we create a relationship which is painful but without growth, the chances are we will recreate the same kind of opportunity until we learn the lesson. Why else do we see some people repeatedly marry actively drinking alcoholics? Or addicts? I believe that until a change comes from *within*, the same kind of partner will manifest over and over again, no matter how different he or she may look on the surface. The answer lies with the *self;* that is the part we need to work on.

Before we can create a healthy, supportive relationship we must first learn how to stand alone. It is critical that we become whole and define ourselves as complete and content *on our own,* before we merge with another human being. Today I realize that I missed a critical step in my adult development because I had never really lived on my own. I went from my parents' home to my marriage. I never learned how to stand on my own two feet and be completely responsible for my own life. I was not a whole person when I got married. How could I have expected to maintain a sense of my own identity when I had never developed a clear idea of who I was by myself?

First, and most important, then, is the commitment to oneself, to one's own journey. It is never right to burden another person with the duty of taking care of us. As soon as we give up our freedom and personal integrity we have lost an essential part of ourselves. Moreover, we run the risk of creating resentment in our beloved. Perhaps Emmanuel says it best: "Relationship is not mutual responsibility. It is mutual love and self-discovery. When two people are bound by more than that, there is servitude and false authority."

It is critical that we learn to love ourselves, nurture and support ourselves. We need to be able to express our inner truth without fear of rejection. Only when we have mastered self-love are we ready to begin the long journey of truly loving our mates, our children, friends and neighbors.

Friends are critical to our well-being in life. I like to say that I have two families. One is my primary family which includes parents, spouse, in-laws, siblings, children, and all other assorted relatives. The other is my family of choice which consists of many caring, committed friends who have become and will remain an integral part of my life. Sometimes my two families mesh and blend; often they are separate. To each family system I make a commitment to maintain our connection and to offer love and support no matter what. We bless each others' lives. Friendship requires nurturing and sharing. I must share who I am honestly and be open to who my friends are as well. I love the message I once read which says, "A friend is someone who accepts me warts and all."

I commit to keeping in touch with my friends, some who reach back to my childhood. I stay in touch (however lightly) with relatives I have not seen for many years. I care about them all and they care about me. Phone calls, birthday cards, Christmas letters, occasional visits keep the ties intact. I have come to understand that there is no separation in spirit though we may be separated by many miles in geography. In prayer and meditation I surround these families with love on a daily basis and by my doing so we all become more strongly connected. The little effort it requires to keep friendships alive is worth more than words can say. I am enriched, supported and cared for as I am willing to reach out to others in my life.

There have been times when my fear has caused me to back away from family and friends. Fear of what? Having to say good-bye? Having to take care of someone? Having to reveal my pain? Having to ask for help? Of losing control? Of having to set boundaries? Of having to disagree? Whatever the fear has been it has limited my experience. The one way to get through the fear is to face it with love and integrity. If I love myself enough to set boundaries, speak my truth and take care of my own needs appropriately, I will be well equipped to have friends.

In order to have friends I must *be* a friend. I need to be willing to be fully *present* in all my friendships and reveal who I truly am. By doing that I empower the people around me to be who they really are. We need to wear no masks of drugs, or self-protection through superficial sharing or humor. When we put on masks such as these, we inhibit real communication. The end result is that we have no *true* friends, just a series of acquaintances who vanish when the painful realities of life intrude as they sometimes do.

Friends and family are our real strength in life, just as relationships (intimate, sexual friendships) can be a real challenge. Somewhere along the way, love and sex got mixed up in our society. The popular media and music are full of images which tell us that sex is the same as love and that dependency will make us happy. We seem to be confused about the whole issue of what we want in relationships. Implied in the messages is that if we find the person who provides us with that magical chemistry of attraction, we are on our way to living happily ever after. After we have had that experience a few times and found out that a good sexual encounter does not mean that we have love, we begin to wonder. Rather than questioning the popular myths, however, we tend to question ourselves and our worthiness as partners. If we already have low self-esteem, we are ripe for self-rejection.

We need to understand that love and sex are two separate issues. Our sexuality is an important component of our humanity. It is the physical, emotional and spiritual expression of ourselves as we were designed to do. Unfortunately, many caregivers suffered sexual abuse as children, whether or not we are fully conscious of that fact. We may not remember, but our bodies remember. If we grew up in dysfunctional families, it follows that we are probably confused about sexuality. Our sexual expression reflects what we believe about ourselves at a deep level, and it's unlikely

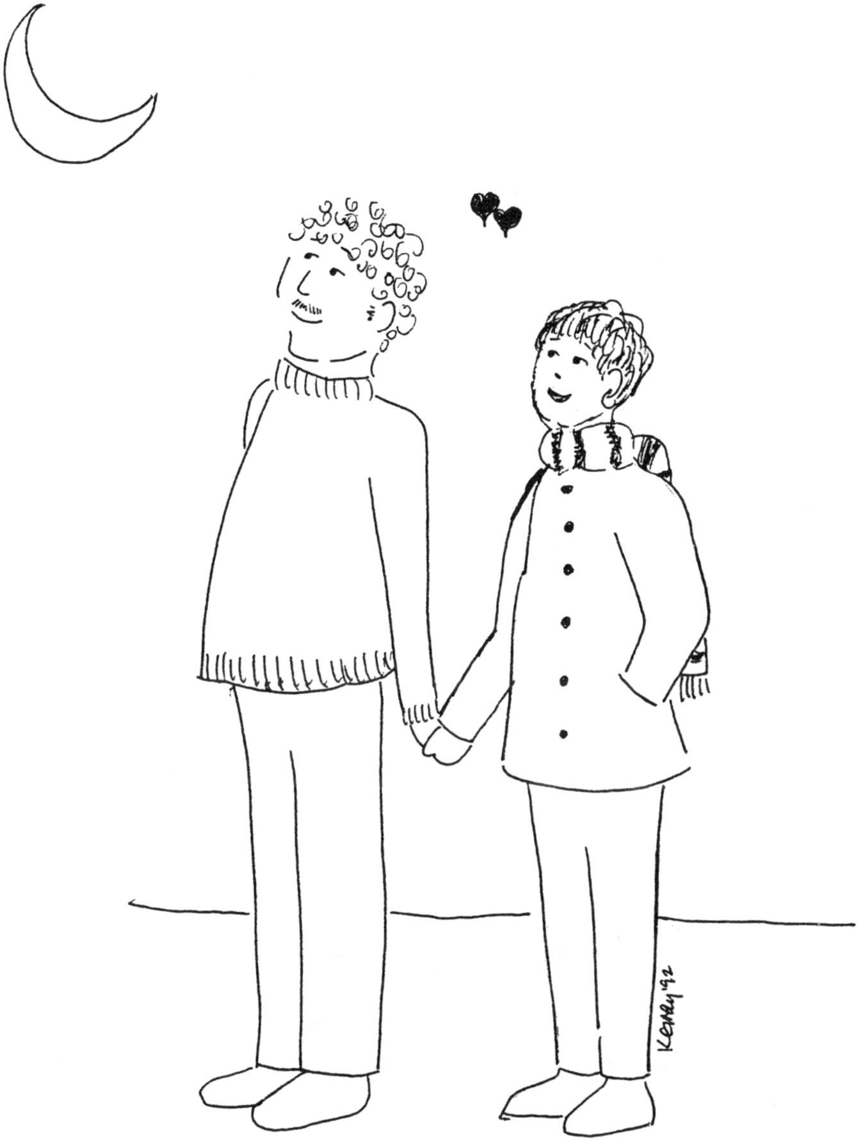

that any dysfunctional family can give children a healthy attitude about who they are.

Many will not acknowledge the importance of sexual self-expression, but according to psychologist Abraham Maslow, sex is one of our basic human needs. He places it in his hierarchy of needs with water, food and shelter. Such needs are difficult to ignore; they must be met before we can move into other levels of expression and accomplishment. Who can write poetry when he is dying of thirst? Is it possible to paint a masterpiece when one's hands are freezing? Can we solve complicated mathematical problems when our bellies are crying out for food? But our sexuality is just as often repressed and ignored, or viewed with fear and suspicion. Many of us were taught that to be sexually active was to be dirty and immoral.

Viewed from a purely physical perspective, sex is a pleasurable experience which brings powerful sensations to the human body. There are few pleasures quite so satisfying to a human being as good sex, either practiced with another or alone. The experience is so pleasant there is the temptation to become addicted to the sensations and spend a disproportionate amount of time in satisfying sexual urges. The physical desires of the body can begin to consume the individual. Relationships may be created which serve only to satisfy the sensual needs of the partners. Other needs are disregarded altogether and the relationship becomes harmful for one or both. Like the gift of fire, sexuality is a beautiful thing that can consume if it be used unwisely.

From an emotional standpoint, sex can create feelings of great joy or infinite pain between partners. It can be soothing and comforting to experience sex with a loving and supportive partner. But there is the potential for the creation of feelings of shame and powerlessness, fear, anger and control. This is why the prospect of physical intimacy can be frightening. Sometimes denying sensuality is easier that dealing with it. From a spiritual point of view, the sexual act can produce a unique sensation of unity between partners which can be matched by no other experience on earth. It is as though the partners join not only with one another, but with the life force of the universe, God himself. No wonder we long to capture such an exquisite feeling of love and recreate it over and over.

I believe what works best is when we have a balance between the physical, emotional and spiritual component of our sexual expression. We must learn how to love ourselves enough to speak our truth about sexual needs and to express them in a way which is loving to ourselves and to our partners. This is not an easy thing to do for most of us.

My experience has been that caregivers find it far easier to please their mates than to please themselves. The time has come for us to understand that in order to be sexually healthy we must be loving and supportive of our needs first. This is not selfish; it is honest. Until we know clearly how to love ourselves and express ourselves honestly and directly, we will not be able to love others in a healthy way. We may be able to use sex as a powerful tool to produce addictions in our partners. They will "need" us, therefore they will stay around. That kind of dependency is not the healthy expression of sexuality. Likewise, if we are hooked into a relationship because we have become addicted to the sex, we are not doing ourselves any favors.

Balanced, well adjusted sexuality implies that because I am a beloved child of God, I am worthy of having a loving, kind, supportive sexual partner who cares very much whether I am satisfied. It means that I can and will say NO to any activity which I feel is dishonest or degrading. It says that I will not be used as a sex object to satisfy the lusts of another being, no matter how positively I feel about him. It says that I have a right to have a happy and fulfilling sex life with a mate who appreciates my uniqueness as a human being. It says that I will not accept treatment which in any ways demeans my humanity. Naturally, it follows that I will honor my chosen partner with the kind of loving kindness which I expect from him.

I never realized until I was divorced that one of the ways my spouse kept me "in my place" was to criticize my body. He often said I could go topless whenever I wanted to since no one would know whether I was a boy or a girl. I laughed along with him when he joked about my flat chest, but I realized later that by keeping me off balance about my lack of physical perfection, he also kept me off balance in other ways, thus defusing my power as a woman. Later I found out in single life that some men are aroused by small breasts, even preferring them to larger ones. One of the first things I did after I was divorced was to throw away my padded bras and learn to love my body as it was, not how some misguided man thought it should be. Sexual put-downs are sexual abuse. Women have suffered sexual abuse for centuries and it is well past time for us to put an end to our acceptance of it.

Women have just as much right to the free expression of their sexuality as men do. There is nothing wrong with adults sharing a totally loving relationship provided it is honest and caring. But there is a lot wrong with using others for one's own pleasure, without any concern for their Inner Being. Persons are not objects. They are spiritual entities who are worthy of respect and honor. Let us remember that when we choose the companions for our journey in life.

We become aware that we are getting better when we notice that our relationships, whatever their nature, are more and more satisfying to us. As we become healthy and more loving to ourselves we automatically attract the same kind of people into our lives. When our self-esteem rises and we learn to set limits for ourselves, we no longer attract companions who abuse and misuse us. The goal is to love ourselves so much we radiate love, acceptance and caring to everyone who comes into our lives. With love of self and others comes peace, contentment and a truly satisfying life.

Today I am married to the kindest, most loving man I have ever known. I waited a long time for him to come into my life. I spent the time studying, learning, experimenting and growing. When I became whole and healthy he arrived. We did not rush into commitment as I had done in my first marriage. We got to know one another and built trust in one another over a period of years. Through him I learned that while I had blamed every man I had ever known for being "emotionally unavailable," *I* had been the one who was more afraid of true intimacy than many of them. We had a small but perfect wedding on the beach in Hawaii, and today we are committed, caring partners in work and in life. I know now that I deserve the kind of love that this wonderful man brings to me daily. For many years I did not.

Of course, the bottom line in real love is commitment, both to the self and others. M. Scott Peck expresses it well when he writes:

Commitment is inherent in any genuinely loving relationship. Anyone who is truly concerned for the spiritual growth of another knows, consciously or instinctively, that he or she can significantly foster that growth only through a relationship of constancy.

When one is willing to really experience life, self, others, and love, the rewards are profound. The beauty and value of love in one's life is perfectly expressed by the philosopher Pierre Teilhard de Chardin:

Love alone is capable of uniting living beings in such a way as to complete and fulfill them, for it alone takes them and joins them by what is deepest in themselves.

WORKBOOK EXERCISE

End of Chapter Eleven

Answer the following questions with "Yes" or "No":

1. I can honestly say that I love myself:

2. It is easy for me to set boundaries in my relationships:

3. I have many friendships with loving, supportive people:

4. I keep in touch with a network of caring family members:

5. I know that I deserve to be in a loving committed relationship:

6. I am in a mutually respectful committed relationship:

7. When things go wrong for me, I am willing to share my pain with people who care about me:

8. I am satisfied with the quality of my sex life:

9. I am "willing to be seen" by my family and friends:

If you have answered "No" to three or more of the above questions, you may find it helpful to do one or more of the following exercises:

1. Make a list of five members of your primary family and commit to being in touch with them by phone or in writing on a weekly basis for the next six weeks.

2. Make a list of three "family of choice" friends and commit to being in touch with them by phone or in writing on a weekly basis for the next six weeks.

3. Make a list of the qualities you want to find in a committed partner. Keep the list in a safe place and read it daily. Become a person who possesses the qualities you admire so that you can draw such a man/woman into your life.

4. Call up someone you have recently met and engage in a conversation. Commit to at least three such phone conversations every week for the next six weeks.

At the end of six weeks make a list of your friends. Examine whether the improvement in your level of inner peace is related to the improvement in your ability to be a friend and to appreciate the friends in your life.

FURTHER READING

Bradshaw, John. *Homecoming: Reclaiming and Championing Your Inner Child.* (Bantam, 1990). Explains how we can heal our relationships as we identify, nurture and heal our own inner child.

Gawain, Shakti. *Living in the Light.* (Whatever Publishing, 1986). A clearly written and engaging book which is very helpful in defining healthy relationships.

Louden, Jennifer. *The Women's Comfort Book.* (Harper, 1992). An excellent resource book to help women develop self-nurturing skills. Lists many ways to get in touch with your needs and to please your body, mind and spirit.

Peck, M. Scott. *The Road Less Travelled: A New Psychology of Love, Traditional Values and Spiritual Growth.* (Simon & Schuster, 1985). Advises us to adhere to a program of self-discipline and love to transform our weaknesses into strengths. The companion workbook volume is *Exploring the Road Less Travelled.*

Ray, Sondra. *Loving Relationships.* (Celestial Arts, 1980). Finding and keeping a perfect mate is easy using this book as a resource and a guide.

Rodegast, Pat, and Stanton, Judith. *Emmanuel's Book.* (Bantam, 1987). A channeled book offering spiritual insight into the meaning of human relationships and many other pertinent questions.

Chapter 12: You're The Boss!

Taking Charge of Your Life

Plant your own garden and decorate your own soul instead of waiting for someone to bring you flowers.

– Anonymous

Care about the approval of others and you will be their prisoner.

– Lao-tzu

I believe that the only way that we can be truly happy in our work is to accept a realistic attitude about what we can and cannot do. We need to learn how to march to the beat of our own drummer, rather than feeling that we are here only to serve and please others. In doing our jobs, we have to learn how to prioritize, how to set limits, how to forgive ourselves if we do not always measure up the way we would like to do. We must allow our imperfections and realize that in fact we are important parts of the picture.

In order for us to love ourselves properly, we must learn how to set boundaries. When others ask us to do more than we think is reasonable we have to state our positions clearly. Often we will be expected to carry a heavier workload than we think is safe. Sometimes we will be asked to work a double shift or double back. On occasion we will be expected to give up a much earned and needed day off. It is all right to say "Yes" to these requests if we truly feel good about doing so. But if we agree in order to please others, trying to fit in, or to be helpful *at our expense,* we are doing a disservice not only to ourselves but to the people around us.

I have rarely met a caregiver who found it easy to refuse a request of any kind. My best approach is to say, "Let me think about it for a while," then give an answer later. I can usually come to a decision that is healthy for me and for other people. The world does not come to an end just because I refuse a request. Amazing, but true.

It is tantalizing to think about the nice fat paycheck which will come as a result of working "doubles" or long hours of overtime. The problem is that having more money does not guarantee greater happiness. We can probably think of many famous (and not so famous) examples which bear this out, and perhaps it is fairest to them not to single out any individuals by name. Suffice to say that having all the money in the world does not necessarily ensure a healthy, balanced life and a sense of serenity.

The ego trap seduces many of us. We begin to feel indispensable to the system when we keep being asked to spend more and more time at work; to give more and more of ourselves at the expense of living a full life on our own. But my experience has taught me that we will be infinitely more satisfied in our work and in our lives when we arrive at a place where we realize that our first responsibility lies with ourselves. I wish I had learned that truth many years ago; I would have been happier much earlier.

We cannot control what others think about us. It is futile to try. We can only do our best to speak our truth as we understand it. If our motives are pure and our lives are lived according to our own high ideals we have nothing to fear. Others will think what they want to. We cannot always please at work, at home, or at play without considering the price we are paying. We will lose in the end. The only time we are sure winners is when we are kind, loving and supportive to ourselves first and then to the people around us.

We must remember that *we* are in charge of our lives. What we are experiencing at any given moment is happening because we create the reality as an opportunity for growth. We are not a victims, and we are not trapped. The only time we are is when we believe we are. We always have choices. The only thing which can really hold us back is our fear, fear of taking charge of our lives, fear of offending, fear of taking a chance, fear of making changes. There is truly nothing to fear. The universe is a safe and benevolent place so long as we believe that it is. We need to have faith in ourselves and our abilities to do whatever it is we want to do. We need to have faith in our Higher Power to direct and support us. With the help of this Power we can create a lives which support our needs perfectly.

We are fortunate in that we have so many choices about our work. With all the choices, however, we must make a commitment. We do not have to limit oursleves to a certain area of health care, though we certainly may. One of my classmates started working in the newborn nursery right after graduation. She is still there more than thirty years later. She has learned so much as the whole area of neonatal care has grown and developed. Such a source of information and expertise she is!

Our work areas may change over the years as our personal goals and interests change. We can commit to caregiving in a general way and follow our bliss as we explore and develop our options. First we need to identify career goals. What exactly do we want to achieve, to master? Professional excellence is a very worthy goal in any area, but it does not mean that we must commit to even a forty-hour work week. Neither does it mean that we commit to any one unit or institution for an entire career. What it does mean is that we need to identify our areas of interest and strengths, and learn and grow into them, at our own pace.

A good practice is to do serious goal-setting every year. The New Year is always an appropriate time for thinking about what we want to accomplish in the next twelve months.

If we don't know our final destination, it is very difficult to plan a sensible journey to get there. We look at what we've accomplished in the past year. This means keeping records of any courses or workshops taken. We then identify what we would like to accomplish in the coming year and write it down. We keep it in a handy spot where it can be referred to at least on a monthly basis. When we are heading in the direction we want to go there is no doubt we will achieve what is desired.

It is exciting to see that many hospitals have well-developed career ladders for staff nurses. I have been a staff nurse in two hospitals which have them. New graduates begin at a clinical level. More experienced RN's are clinical II's. Those who would like to develop a broader area of clinical responsibility work to become level III RN's. The goal is to provide opportunities for staff nurses to advance without having to leave the bedside. With more responsibility comes more pay and the opportunity for professional growth. Of course it is a lot more work, but the level III nurses I know truly enjoy it. They may assist with management in their unit, but their primary function is role modeling top-notch clinical practice, and they are very good at it. Many service professionals enjoy the challenge of clinical ladders for career growth, e.g. social workers, counselors.

Another real opportunity for growth and networking is to become involved in your professional organization. You can be very active or you can serve in a minor but needed function. There is great power and inspiration in joining together with our peers to create change and growth. Many side benefits can come as a result of professional networking. Getting involved with the leaders in your field may inspire other ways to grow, such as getting more education.

When I began my career as a nurse I never dreamed that I would someday choose to go back to college and get my baccalaureate degree. Like most diploma RN's of that era, I felt that a degree was a bit superfluous. But there came a time when I realized it was necessary. If I wanted to pursue a satisfying career with as many options as possible, I would need to have that BSN after my name. I made a commitment to two more years of college. I maintained a work schedule of twenty-four hours a week and managed to take care of home and family as well. It was a lot of work. Perhaps at some level I understood that there would be major changes coming in my life and the degree would be important for my success.

Going back to school at the age of forty-three was not easy, but it was oh, so liberating. I would strongly urge any person who is interested in doing so to go for it. I felt like a dried up old sponge that has just fallen into a bucket of water. I totally expanded in every way. It was a truly life-changing and life-enhancing experience for me. I developed more self-confidence, assertiveness and growth than I ever thought possible.

It was fascinating to me to find out how much more control I had over my life when I had more education. Having reached my goal of completing my degree, I was now ready to return to nursing management and see if my skills had given me any more power to manage my life. The last time I had gone into management I burned out. This time was very different. Now I understood the theory; with new tools at my disposal I was able to take a troubled nursing unit and turn it into one which was a model for others in the hospital. One vice-president referred to me as "the shining star in the management crown" at that institution. Goal setting indeed worked for me, and it was well worth the effort.

For those interested in nursing management, there are many opportunities in that area. We can learn more about management theory, then practice by offering to work more charge. We can go back to school, or read management journals and books about management. There are many, many ways in which to develop natural talents in that area.

We may need to be willing to move to a different unit in the hospital, or a different hospital. Or even be open to the possibility of relocating to a different part of the country. As they say, the sky is the limit!

I so admired a woman who was in my BSN class when I went back to school. She had a full-time job as the nurse manager of a large and busy neonatal unit in a very progressive hospital. She took extra classes for years, working towards her degree. As soon as she finished her BSN she began to work on her Master's in business. Her goal was to become a division manager in her hospital. She has accomplished it. In addition to her work and school efforts, she has also handled a large home and family. Joan is only one of the amazing nurses I have known. What makes the difference for these exceptional individuals is that they are clear about their goals and systematically work towards them, as Joan did. Some drift and float along expecting that we will get to a destination that we have not even bothered to identify.

The setting of goals in the professional area in not the only one which is important. Another area where we must learn to be assertive and responsible is in the setting of financial goals. A current fact of life is that most North American women will spend at least twenty-five years in the work force. Because of high demand, health professionals are more fortunate than many in that we have many choices about how, when, where and how long to work. We are earning more money now than ever before. Perhaps it is time to become more competent in handling it.

There are many fine books on the subject of financial management. There are classes, seminars and workshops which are available. There are many professionals who make their living by advising people on the wise use of their financial resources. Perhaps the best way to find a good one to help us is to talk to friends and the friends of our parents. Find out who they use for accounting, stocks & bonds, and investments. We can meet the people they recommend and then make our choices. We must choose carefully and not give up total control of financial matters to any one individual. The media are full of stories of well-known persons who let exactly this happen, with disastrous results. We must pay attention to the money we earn, and even the money received as gifts. Money is like a child: we created it and need to take care of it. We can't wait for someone else to "save" us.

It is up to us as individuals to take charge of every area of our lives, and not only the financial. It is about being powerful and assertive; it is about developing the masculine aspect of ourselves. Most of the caregivers I know have well cultivated the feminine aspect of themselves. We are expert about being nurturing, intuitive, receptive and kind. We do need to develop the masculine, ambitious, mechanical, intrusive, take-charge part of ourselves. We have the ability to manage our own resources when we are willing to take charge and do so. The not so well known truth is that much of the money in North America is controlled by women.

Managing our lives in a way which is satisfying to us is our own responsibility. One thing which needs some degree of our management is our relationship to the institution where we work. Most of us realize that we are part of a very imperfect health care system. Certainly, the system provides some of the finest technological services in the world. I do not argue with this fact. But the demand for more and more technology to save fewer and fewer patients is strange indeed. Where else in the world are heart, liver, kidney, and lung transplants commonplace? Where else are there dozens of medications - nearly all exorbitantly expensive - for the alteration of every part of every body system?

Perhaps we need to take a critical and courageous look at the entire structure. We call it a health care system but in truth it is almost entirely geared toward the care of the sick. Appallingly little is done to promote wellness and prevent illness and injury. This present health care system accounts for more than twelve percent of the U.S. gross national product in this complex economy. A staggering number of dollars being spent each minute of every day. Even with all the expenditures, Americans are not substantially healthier than we were before, though we are living more years. Many, many people cannot afford any health care at all. We spend enormous amounts of money on saving the life of one premature infant and are unwilling to invest in good prenatal care and teaching of poor pregnant women to prevent prematurity problems.

A strange situation indeed! We caregivers are caught in the middle. Many administrators complain bitterly about the high cost of professional staff. As a result, they cut corners, overload their professionals and create dangerous work situations where the patient is at risk. The caregiver is constantly on the edge of burnout. Many letters in Ann Landers' newspaper column attest to this fact. Caregivers in many parts of the country are leaving the profession in large numbers, yet many bottom-line oriented hospital administrators refuse to deal with the problem.

It may well be that some hospitals need to close their doors if they are unable to give the kind of care which their patients deserve and are certainly paying for. Nurses and other health care professionals must speak out. If we find ourselves in situations where overload threatens the safety of our patients or clients, we must take action. We need to confront supervisors. If managers are unwilling or unable to take action, we can follow up with letters to administration. Strikes are not out of the question. The ultimate goal is to provide for the safe care of our patients. When it becomes impossible for us to do that, we need to do something about it. After all, our primary role is that of patient advocate. We must also be advocates for ourselves. Caregivers may have to become free agents and select the places where they are willing to work. Some do this by becoming independent professionals through private agencies. This approach works well for many individuals.

There are many fine institutions for taking care of the sick. Some are better than others at recognizing and supporting their caregivers. A few have no problems retaining and motivating staff. And in each institution there are many different departments. It *is* possible to find a spot which feels really good. One must be positive and creative in the search. We need to be willing to make job changes until the fit is right. Ultimately we *can* find the best spot for us.

Having said all that about taking charge of our lives and being responsible for ourselves, I am going to add another dimension to this whole area. While it is true that we need to "jump through hoops" in order to comply with the way that our society works, there is a larger picture. Even though we must do certain things in order to be "in the world," such as get a good education, prepare a resume, apply for a job, perform well on that job, collect a paycheck and be responsible for what we do with our money, we ultimately have a far greater power available to us should we choose to use it.

This power is the creative force within us which can produce miracles if we tune into it and use it for the highest good. We are indeed spiritual beings having a human experience. If we remain in the human part of the experience and believe that we have no control over what happens to us, that is exactly what we will get. Most human beings on this planet think that way. As we think, so we create, so we are.

I invite you to consider another way of being in the world. That is the way of acknowledging our inner power and hooking into it in a conscious and purposeful way. We can create abundance far more easily than most of us realize. We need to practice three main principles in order to manifest prosperity and power in our lives.

Principle One: The first principle is that we need to GIVE THANKS FOR WHAT WE HAVE NOW. The truth is that nearly everyone in the Western world lives a whole lot better than everyone else on the planet. How can we not be thankful? No matter how much more of anything we would like to have, we will be happier, more peaceful and more aware of how well we live if we take the time to give thanks for everything. I sometimes get into fear of lack, especially when I am stepping into unknown territory of a new job or new place to live or a new project which may or may not succeed. I make a practice of being thankful, even as I pay the bills down to the last dollar in my bank account. I am so glad that there are people and businesses out there that provide the goods and services that I need and I appreciate their having trust in my commitment to pay them for their services.

Principle Two: The second principle of creating abundance is to AFFIRM AND VISUALIZE IT constantly. No more thinking about what we have not. We focus on what is true about us, that we are beloved children of a benevolent father/mother God. As such, we are entitled to all abundance in every area of our lives. I make a practice of doing affirmations on a daily basis, especially when I find myself slipping back into the old fear modes of limited thinking. I carry a stack of index cards when I go running or walking and read them out loud, focusing intently on getting the belief deep down into my subconscious mind where it can get to work. Doing this on a daily basis is one of the most powerful ways I know to create any kind of change in my life. Many other people have found this to be true as well.

Some examples of affirmations for abundance that I use are:

I AM WORTHY OF FINANCIAL ABUNDANCE

I AM WORTHY OF SUCCESS

I AM WORTHY OF A CAREER THAT I LOVE.

I HAVE A PERFECT RIGHT TO $ ABUNDANCE $.

WORTHINESS IS MY DIVINE NATURE.

PROSPERITY IS MY BIRTHRIGHT AS A CHILD OF GOD.

We need to realize that having abundance and power in our lives is part of the principle of creative thinking. Whether or not we realize it, we are creating our reality every time we focus on a thought or hold a belief about ourselves or the world. When we are conscious of how we think, we begin to be aware of how limiting - or powerful - our thinking can be. For example, I had a period of time in my life when I slipped into the idea of lack. When I received my paycheck and sat down to pay the bills I kept thinking about how big the bills were and how little money I had to pay them. Each payday, I would make myself miserable about the "problems" I was having with not enough money. As I continued to focus on "not enough" it seemed that there was less and less money to do the job. When I look back I realize how very silly that was because I HAD EVERYTHING I NEEDED in order to be happy in the moment. I had what was necessary and the lack was produced only by my limited thinking.

Principle Three: What I did was to give thanks when I paid the bills and be genuinely grateful for all my blessings. And then I began to learn one of the best-kept secrets of the ages. This is the third and probably most powerful yet least understood principle of creating abundance. We need to SHARE WHAT WE HAVE ON A REGULAR BASIS. I read the writings of Catherine Ponder who teaches her beliefs about the blessings of tithing or sharing one tenth of one's income with the source of spiritual strength. I began to give the first ten percent of my income to several spiritual, charitable and earth-supportive organizations. I blessed each check as I wrote and mailed it. Then I paid the regular bills.

The result was more abundance for me! It was amazing. I had changed nothing but my attitude and suddenly I had more money and more blessings than ever. I have continued this practice because it works. It helps me to share what I have with others every bit as much as it works for them. We all make a difference in the world, every one of us who wakes up to the real source of our power and abundance. Everything comes from a loving God, everything. In order to be happy we simply stop and pay attention to what is true. It is this: WHEN WE GIVE TO OTHERS WE ARE REALLY GIVING TO OURSELVES!

One of the most generous people I know is Judy. She is another one of us caregivers. What others have struggled to learn, she has always known: that it blesses her as much as it blesses others when she shares what she has. She was generous and giving as a child and has remained so. She is the original worthy recipient of that time-worn phrase, "she would give you the shirt off her back." It is true. She gives away more things and money than any person I know. She doesn't think about it and there is no ego involved, she just does it out of love and concern for others. As a result, she is continually blessed with a flow of supply that is sometimes quite amazing. It is as though the universe uses her for a conduit and she is never in a space of financial lack. She enjoys abundance, "filled up, pressed down and running over."

Finally, taking charge of our lives means that we give up forever the idea that we are victims. Our life is exactly what we want it to be, whether or not we are willing to be accountable for that fact. We are just as powerful and positive and prosperous as we are willing to be, no more, no less. It is up to us.

We can practice taking responsibility for ourselves by saying things like:

Iwant .... **I don't want** ....

I need .... **I don't need** ....

I expect .... **I don't expect** ....

I like .... **I don't like** ....

If you are anything like me, taking charge of your own life and every part of it has not been easy. We caregivers seem to be so reluctant to take care of ourselves. We limit our abundance and we limit our experience. We seem to think we have no other choice. We are learning to do better. I am seeing more and more self-love showing up in the actions of caregivers I know. We are learning that we are worthy of having lives that we love. Why not? We deserve it! We are a pretty wonderful bunch of people.

WORKBOOK EXERCISE

End of Chapter Twelve

Answer the following questions with "Yes" or "No".

1. I am well satisfied with my present job:

2. I am able to set limits on the amount of time I spend at work:

3. I have no reason to complain about my job situation:

4. I have a well thought-out plan for retirement:

5. My savings plan is well organized:

6. I think my boss and my institution really appreciate me:

7. I take good care of myself:

8. I have a good idea of my professional goals for the next five years:

9. I have learned and grown a lot professionally in the past year:

If you answered "No" to three or more questions, you may want to do some serious evaluation of your job satisfaction and your goals for professional growth. It will help you to do one or all of the following exercises, depending on your vision of what your needs are

1. Meet with a peer/colleague who could serve as a good role model for you. Ask for her/his assistance in evaluating and setting goals for professional growth.

2. Read one of the suggested books for inspiration on taking charge of your life. Make a list of specific measurable goals for changing your life and the way you manage it. Then do it.

3. Meet with a certified financial planner for some advice on goal setting and money management. Many financial institutions provide this service free of charge.

There, now don't you feel more in charge of your life?

FURTHER READING

Chaney, Casey. *Ready, Willing, and Terrified.* (Mocha Publishing, 1991). Concise, well-organized method for creating change in one's life.

Ponder, Catherine. *The Dynamic Laws of Prosperity.* (De Vorss, 1962). A metaphysical approach to creating financial abundance.

Porter, Sylvia. *Sylvia Porter's Your Finances in the 1990s.* (Prentice-Hall, 1990).

Roman, Sanaya, and Packer, Duane. *Creating Money.* (H.J. Kramer, 1988). Another spiritual approach to money and finances.

VanCaspel, Venita. *Money Dynamics for the 1990s.* (Simon & Schuster, 1988).

Chapter 13: Journey Into Light

Acknowledging Our Spirituality

This is the message of religious teachings in both East and West: seek spiritual values first, whatever is tangibly needed will follow after.

– Jean Shinoda Bolen

We have the power of choice - we may follow the magic path of intuition, or the long hard road of experience, by following the reasoning mind.

– Florence Scovell Shinn

I do not speak against religion. I question the use of dogma. To believe in the God in everyone is the ultimate religion. It does not matter what path you take to get there.

– Emmanuel

The spiritual journey is really the only road there is. Mine began many long years ago, of that I am sure. I have felt very close to God ever since I was a small child. He has always been a God of great love, compassion and forgiveness to me, no matter what anyone else told me about Him. Never have I viewed God as angry, vengeful or cruel. He is the source of all my strength, comfort, hope and happiness. Nothing in this world would have any meaning to me without God.

However, my perception of God has changed. The realization about God's presence in nature came to me very vividly as I walked in the beautiful Sonora desert around Tucson. The peace and loveliness of that place spoke to me of the eternal; of the infinite glory around us all the time. I saw

God manifesting as the magnificent palo-verde tree in its full golden blooms of springtime. God was everywhere, in everything, all around me. I could not escape His presence. As I walked I talked to Him. I cried. I listened. I grew and learned. I felt a sense of peace and destiny which truly overwhelmed me with love. I often thought about the wonderful movie *Fiddler on the Roof* when I talked to God. The character Tevye did that too. God became more real and present for me. I held nothing back. I learned that I was loved, supported and cherished beyond all human understanding.

That time was one of great personal anguish for me as I dealt with the reality of my separation and divorce. I felt the pain fully and moved through it with God's help. There was no turning back. Later I came to understand that God manifests as human. I realized when I watched the exquisite performance of *Swan Lake* by the San Francisco ballet company. I suddenly understood that the grace and power of the dancers was God manifesting through human beings. I saw that the gorgeous costumes had been created by God through the dedicated designers and seamstresses. The gifted musicians were bringing forth music which caused my heart to pound with the thrill of it. They too were manifesting God on the earth plane. Every person who played a part in that production was doing it. As they followed their creative potential and developed talents they were manifesting the God within.

It does not matter what line of work we choose, or where we choose to do it. If we are truly doing what we love and loving what we do, we are co-creators with the Infinite Power of the Universe. It is clear to me that if we dedicate ourselves to our best performance, lovingly completed, each day, we are manifesting God. As a nurse, I manifest God, just as you do. I did not always understand that, but I do today.

Every caregiver can relate many stories from her own career which clearly indicate that she was a critical or change agent for someone at some time. Many such experiences have come to me when I least expected them. Afterward I have had such sense of humble gratitude that I was the instrument which God used in order to assist one of my brothers and sisters on earth.

The amazing thing is that when we bless others by manifesting the God within, we cannot help but heap blessing on ourselves as well. The joy and peace which come to us when we sense that we have truly made a difference for a fellow human being is so immense as to defy description. Ask any caregiver. It is the reason we came into our professions and, despite our many frustrations and difficulties, it is the main reason we stay.

Our Higher Self is in complete charge of the human experience. It has all the knowledge of what it is we came here to accomplish this time. If we get in touch with that part of ourselves, we will have lives which are infinitely happier, more serene and more productive than we ever thought possible. The secret lies in getting quiet and paying attention to the Voice within.

At first the Voice is very quiet and sometimes difficult to hear. The more we listen, however, the more clear and powerful it becomes. As we develop the ability to use that inner guidance system in every aspect of our daily lives, we get into full harmony with the flow of the universe. Peace is possible. Commitment to a higher, more creative course is possible. Serenity becomes a way of life.

Everyone can remember instances when she had an inner knowing about something. If she failed to honor that wisdom, she said later, "Oh, I knew I should have stopped to check this or that. I had a feeling." Or we are prompted to make a telephone call and the shared communication turns out to be very important to one or both parties.

I recall receiving a phone call from a friend when I was debating about whether or not I should move to Hawaii. I really did not want to leave my home and friends in Tucson, but I felt compelled to explore this new opportunity. I was thinking very hard about the decision, uncertain about what to do. When Samantha called she said, "I don't know why, I just feel like I need to get in touch with you. What is going on?" When I told her how I was agonizing about my decision she said: "Well, just consider it an invitation from the Universe. You can accept it or reject it. It's up to you." Oddly enough, that statement was all I needed to hear in order to clarify my thought.

I decided to accept the invitation and set the wheels in motion, realizing that if it was the right move for me, everything would fall into place perfectly. If not, nothing I could do would make it turn out right. One by one, every obstacle to my leaving fell away, and quickly. Within a very short time I had found a good renter for my house, a job in Honolulu, money for the trip and all the encouragement and support I ever needed to make the big move.

By paying attention to her inner Voice, my friend was able to save me a great deal of struggle. She listened; she acted on her intuition and I needed to hear what she had to say. This sort of thing happens again and again as we become more open and sensitive to the Inner Direction.

A story comes to mind as I reflect on this principle. I once had the experience of disregarding my inner Voice when it strongly urged me to go to the little hospital where I was working as the director of nurses. My family and I were on our way to Easter sunrise service which started at six a.m. As we drove into the town from our home in the country I had a compelling urge to stop at the hospital because "something is wrong there". I thought about having my husband drop me off but decided that I was being foolish. Even though there were only two staff on the night shift, both were capable people as was our doctor on call. When we drove by the hospital I could see no evidence of undue activity outside the building, no extra cars or ambulances, so I said nothing to my family as we passed. Later that day I learned that there had been a terrible crisis.

For the first time in the history of our town there had been an attempted murder. The patient was an elderly lady who had been brutally attacked by a young man. He had slipped into her home during the night, beaten and raped her and left her for dead. Her friends found her when they stopped to pick her up for the church service. She survived the initial trauma but eventually died. Though the staff had managed the situation very well, my presence would have helped enormously. My being there would not have made a difference in her survival, but it could have helped in the frantic attempt the staff needed to carry out in order to stabilize her condition. The truth was that I knew in my heart that something was very wrong that day and I did not listen to my inner Voice. It was a powerful and helpful lesson for me. Today I listen carefully to that sixth sense and I follow its message.

When we stop to think about it, we can all tell many tales of having ignored our intuition and later realizing our mistake. The trick is to start really paying attention to our God part. That part of us has all knowledge and wisdom and will never lead us astray. It may tell us things we disregard or do not want to hear, but it will never lie. It is just a sort of feeling which is somewhere in the middle of our stomach. We can't describe it, but it really is there and we know it. The more we listen to it, the louder and clearer it gets until it is the moment by moment director of our lives.

There are some wonderful books being published today which can help us to get in touch with our spirituality. The writings of Shirley MacLaine are a well-known example. One may or may not agree with her individual beliefs, but it is impossible not to admire her courage for sharing the story of her spiritual journey in a series of books. She took a tremendous risk when she went public with her message, but in doing so, she has stimulated the search by countless others.

It was the reading of her books which started me on my journey. I don't always enjoy her writing style, but I love her honesty. She has fearlessly revealed the truth about her quest. She tells about how she went to metaphysical bookstores to find what she needed. At times books fairly leapt into her hands. I have followed that path, and the truth is that "when the student is ready, the teacher appears." It seems that when the Universe sees that you are genuinely ready to learn, you will be provided with exactly what you need to assist in the experience.

Another teacher who has helped many to start their search is Shakti Gawain. Her book *Creative Visualization* has sold two million copies worldwide and was followed by her *Living in the Light*. There are many such writers today. Dr. Wayne Dyer's books are a great help to many. I was given a copy of his *You'll See it When You Believe It,* and I found myself underlining about a fourth of the text! It all rang so true for my Inner Being. I believe that readers of these and similar volumes are hungry for the wisdom these teachers can share with us.

One of my favorite spiritual writers is Alan Cohen. He has many publications to his credit now and each one is a gift. He has such a joyful way of sharing his wisdom with the reader that it is a pleasure to learn from him. I have heard him speak and he radiates love and peace.

Even spirits are writing books these days, by channeling through humans. The first such book that I read was *You Are God,* by Mary. I don't know who Mary is, but she introduced the book by saying that since they were not her words, she could not take credit for them by having her surname on the cover. I love *Emmanuel's Book;* it feels like truth and goodness. The books by Orrin and DaBen are also enlightening and satisfying.

A Course in Miracles is a widely known set of teachings which has also come through from the other side in recent years. It contains great wisdom for healing our world. The story of how the books came into being through the work of Helen Schucman and William Thetford is fascinating and is recalled in the book, *Journey Without Distance*. Helen refused to have her name as the author of *Course in Miracles* because she recognized that it was clearly not her writing. She was simply the instrument for the creation.

It seems that as mankind becomes more willing to explore spirituality (as opposed to dogma), the higher level beings are more able to come in and assist us in our efforts. We are beginning to raise our consciousness to the truth of our divinity. When we look at the teachings of all the great masters such as Jesus and Buddha, we can see how very congruent the new age ideas are. Truth is truth. All religions started out with the essence of Truth. Alas, man has felt compelled to use his intellect to alter and modify it.

For example, I am told there were once many references to reincarnation in the Bible. Over time they have been deleted by the men who were copying the texts, or by various church councils who decided that they were not acceptable teachings. I believe in the idea of reincarnation. It just feels right to me. I know about several of my past lives. We all have the knowledge of all our past lives within us; we need only to access it. I never have accepted that death was the end of anything, only a transition from one level to another. Birth and death are similar processes, sometimes difficult but always necessary.

My favorite true story suggesting reincarnation is about a little boy, three years old. His mother had just brought home a new baby and the child wanted to go into the bedroom to "talk to her." The mother was understandably anxious about permitting him to go into the room alone, but she did allow it. Waiting, outside the bedroom door, she was moved to tears when she heard her son say to the baby: "Tell me about God. I am beginning to forget."

A friend shared another experience along that line. She was with a group of young mothers who were engrossed in discussion about childbirth while their little ones played about the room. One woman began to cry as she told about a stillborn child she had had two years prior to the birth of her little boy who was sitting at her feet. The child put his arms around her and said: "Don't cry, mommy. That was me and I'm here now."

The idea of karma is one which I can easily accept today. All it means is that in the upward evolutionary journey towards higher consciousness, we need to balance things. We choose how we will do it; it is not punishment for past misdeeds. Sin is simply error or ignorance of truth. When the soul leaves the earth plane it has the opportunity to examine that lifetime and decide how to continue its growth. It may choose any way it wishes in order to continue learning. There is free will in the universe; we may choose good or evil and then get to determine how to balance out what we have experienced.

For me, karma explains many things which I have found puzzling in the past. Why is there child abuse? Why do some people seem to have to suffer so much in this life? How is it that some seem to rise above tragedy and grow into brighter beings? If we think about suffering as opportunity to evolve to higher levels of consciousness, it all makes perfect sense. I don't believe that mankind will have to learn all lessons this way forever. There is a higher awareness evolving, and rapidly, on this planet. Some day we will see a world of peace and harmony, where there is no more need for sickness, famine, pain or strife.

My new understanding about spirituality, karma and life lessons has helped me enormously in my nursing practice. I once railed against the kind of suffering which I witnessed.

No longer. I now understand that the human spirit is in charge of everything that happens to it and even if I don't understand the value of someone else's life experience, it is perfect for their growth at this time.

I recently met a beautiful woman patient who had had a devastating accident. She was left paralyzed from the neck down and will spend the rest of her life in a wheelchair. As I worked with her, we talked about the changes which will have to occur in her life, her relationships and her whole world. She accepts that she can handle what has come her way. She is surrounded by a loving, supportive family, and she has many helpful and kind-hearted friends. She has no real financial concerns. She has never before had a serious, life-threatening challenge, and she is optimistic that she will be able to master this one. I believe her. I support her and encourage her to live her life fully, productively and yes, even happily, in her new body state. She will do it beautifully, I know. I see this as a wonderful opportunity for her to evolve spiritually and to teach everyone around her as she grows. These are life lessons for all of us, as well as for the patient.

My attitude toward this amazing woman was one of acceptance for her inner choice. Of course on a conscious level, we humans would never choose such a difficult way to learn and grow, but at a spiritual level, what a perfect chance to evolve! I love and support her on her journey.

Unfortunately, it was not so easy for my younger nursing colleagues to deal with our patient's experience. One young nurse came out of her room feeling quite devastated and sorrowful about the patient's situation. I understood. I once felt the same way in the face of the extraordinarily difficult places in which I have found many of my patients. I now understand that this is an opportunity for growth for this woman and for her family. I have full confidence that they will be okay, though their road may be a hard one. Of course, I do not tell patients that is what I see them doing. Most are not ready to see that and it would only cause them distress to think that they had willed what had happened to them. But it really is their journey, their karma, their choice. There are no accidents, of that I am sure.

When we, as caregivers, have a strongly developed sense of our spirituality, we are empowered to handle the most difficult situations with equanimity. We can accept. We can detach and we can walk with our patients along the paths they have chosen. We can trust that all is well, though it does not appear to be at times. We have a Higher Power guiding our footsteps and so does each and every one of the humans we encounter on the journey.

I said to the man who stood at the Gate of the Year, "Give me a light that I might tread safely into the unknown." And he replied, "Go out into the darkness and put your hand into the hand of God. That shall be to you better than light and safer than a known way."

– Minnie Louise Haskins
(Quoted by King George VI in his Christmas Broadcast, 1939)

WORKBOOK EXERCISE

End of Chapter Thirteen.

Answer the following questions "Yes" or "No":

1. I am able to see and acknowledge a deeper meaning in life:

2. No matter what difficulties my patients/clients encounter, I can remain caring but detached:

3. I have often noticed my intuition at work in my life:

4. I always honor my Inner Voice when I get in touch with it:

5. I remain serene despite being in the midst of chaos and suffering at times:

6. I connect with my Higher Power on a regular basis:

7. I get much comfort from my association with my spiritual support group, church, synagogue or other religious body:

8. I get inspiration and hope from reading spiritual works:

9. I feel a sense of the presence of God when I am out in nature:

10. I have noticed God at work in my life:

If you have answered "No" to three or more of the above questions you may wish to complete the following exercises:

1. Read one or more of the suggested books at the end of this chapter.

2. Make a practice of time alone outdoors for at least two hours once a week. Pay attention to your surroundings. Be still.

3. Talk to someone who seems very peaceful and happy in his or her life. Find out about their spiritual journey.

There is no more interesting discovery than the one into the realm of spiritual Truth. Peace is the great reward.

FURTHER READING

Bolen, Jean Shinoda. *The Tao of Psychology: Synchronicity and the Self*. (Harper & Row, 1979). Explains the concept that there are no accidents, and provides guidance on recognizing the signals in your own life and seeing the divine connection.

Cohen, Alan. *The Dragon Doesn't Live Here Anymore*. (Alan Cohen Publications, 1981). Lighthearted, inspiring book for those who want to incorporate spirituality into their everyday living.

Hay, Louise. *You Can Heal Your Life*. (Hay House, 1984). Classic New Age text looks at all illness as being caused by disharmony of emotion and spirit, and shows how we can heal ourselves by correcting our view of the world.

MacLaine, Shirley. *Going Within*. (Bantam, 1989). One of the best of Maclaine's books on her spiritual quest. Subjects covered in this volume include spiritual healers, psychic surgeons, channellers, and the body's energy centers. Other titles in the series include *Out on a Limb* and *Dancing in the Light*.

Roman, Sanaya. *Spiritual Growth: Being Your Higher Self*. (H.J. Kramer, 1989). A channeled book designed to help people move onward on the spiritual path, giving practical tools to do so.

Siegel, Bernie. *Love, Medicine & Miracles: Lessons Learned About Self-Healing from a Surgeon's Experience with Exceptional Patients.* (Harper, 1986). Explores the concept that we create our own illnesses, and that we can cure ourselves by changing negative thought patterns.

Zukav, Gary. *The Seat of the Soul.* (Simon & Schuster, 1989). A blend of Eastern mysticism, quantum physics and other metaphysical ideas by the author of *The Dancing Wu Li Masters.*

Chapter 14: Letting Go

When Death is the Issue

To everything there is a season,
A time for every purpose under heaven:
A time to be born,
And a time to die.

Ecclesiastes 3: 1-2

In order for us caregivers to be effective in our roles, we must be spiritually healthy and well balanced. It is important to our patients/clients and it is critical for our own survival in our professions. I do not mean that we must be religious, nor that we try to persuade anyone to accept our own particular philosophy about the important issues in our human experience. The truth is that we cannot help others accept their reality until we have formulated a comfortable concept about the meaning of life and death for ourselves.

One way that my own spiritual growth has helped me in my nursing practice is in the way I deal with the issue of death and dying. In the many years that I have been in nursing, I have been with many people as they made their final journey and transition. Like most of my peers, I was at first uncomfortable working with dying patients. I will never forget the first time I witnessed a death and the terror I felt when I had to prepare the body for the morgue. Like most young people, I had never encountered death before. My questions when I began were like everyone else's: "What do I say to this young person who is suffering from a terminal illness?" "How can I be of help to a family who has just lost a beloved child?" The reason I had trouble was mainly because I had not yet become comfortable with the idea of my own mortality. Now I am very much aware that death is a natural and normal event, much like birth. There is nothing to dread or fear. It is only a transition from one level of reality to another.

In most of the world's cultures, the family and friends surround, nurture and support the person who is leaving the earth. They show their appreciation, love and respect for the natural cycle of life. The dying are not left alone. Their families do not have to struggle and grieve by themselves. Dying members are not taken away from their homes and placed in an unfamiliar and uncomfortable environment. Children are included in the process and come to understand that death is a natural part of life. The funeral rites provide an opportunity to mourn openly and then to celebrate the life of the deceased. Life has its own rhythms; it goes on.

In many of the world's cultures, the dying process is handled very much like the birth event. Everyone gathers together and supports the family which is in transition. In our country we are finally learning how to view childbirth as a natural, normal event. This has made a great improvement in the way human infants make their entry into our world. We are learning how to be more tribal and supportive of the family which is changing form. But in the area of leaving the planet, we "civilized" people have a great deal to learn.

Ours is the only culture in the world which views death as a failure. Our medical technology has become so highly advanced that we can literally prolong life indefinitely. I have seen this happen time and time again, and it can be disturbing. Recently I read a newspaper article which stated that it is better to choose a large, metropolitan, teaching hospital for your care when you are sick. The only criterion for making this claim is that once admitted, fewer people die in the big institutions. It is assumed that *any* kind of life at all is better than death. That is a very strange position to take. Many doctors view the death of one of their patients as an indication that as professionals, they have missed the mark. Somehow, the death of a patient is associated with their egos about medical expertise. Like the rest of the members of all the health care teams, doctors need to come to grips with their own ideas of mortality and the meaning of life and death. When they have failed to do that, they have a very difficult time allowing a patient to die with peace and dignity.

Another point to remember is that in our society many individuals and companies make a lot of money keeping people alive. The quality of life does not seem to matter. I have seen the frail elderly admitted to intensive care units and put on respirators when they have little hope of survival and no chance of returning to a high quality of life. They are put on complex internal monitoring systems and given great numbers of expensive drugs. Their care costs are in the hundreds of thousands of dollars per admission. I think many persons would be shocked to think that perhaps one reason that their loved ones are being so tenderly cared for at such great cost is simple greed. I do not say that greed is a conscious motivator any more than the physician's professional vanity is something of which he is aware. But these are very real factors in our confused medical system, and we need to be honest about that.

Another problem is that so many of us are unwilling to face the reality of the inevitable experience. We do little to prepare for death; we do not discuss it openly in families or with doctors. The sentiment goes something like: if I do not think about it, death will not happen to me. It was okay to take that illusory attitude in the days before all of our modern technology was developed. But it is not all right today. We need to be clear about preferences on the issue of artificial life support before we have a health crisis. The families who have talked about sickness and death and decided what they want are usually spared the agony of decision-making during that event.

When my sixty-three year old mother found out that she had extensive carcinoma and could expect to live only a short time, she and my step-father were prepared. They had talked about the issue and had both decided that they wanted no heroics. Mom declined her doctor's suggestion that she undergo extensive chemotherapy. He was upset with her decision, even though he could not assure her of either a longer life or a tolerable quality of life if she agreed to his treatment program. We supported her beliefs. It was clearly her body, her choice and her life. I told her the truth about patients I had taken care of who had the same diagnosis. She deserved to get honest answers to all her questions and she did. From the time of her diagnosis to the day of her death she had exactly one month to live. And live she did. She told her friends what was happening and asked for their support. Her family members all came to say good-bye. She played cards with her bridge club. She did everything that she wanted to do. While she was alive, she received the visits, flowers, gifts and prayers of everyone who loved her. There were so many. With great care, she planned her own funeral. Her main problem was pain control and she managed that well at home until just a few days before she died.

My mother created her own reality when she refused to accept someone else's decision for her life. She told her doctor that she would rather spend her last days enjoying the time she had left rather than suffering with nausea and vomiting and "watching my hair fall out." The quality of her last days on earth was wonderful for her and for us. Of course we did not want her to leave but it would have been selfish to hold her back. She was ready. She made the very best of each moment until she drew her last breath.

I will never forget that night. She was comatose and we were all gathered around her hospital bed. My big, macho step-brother surprised us all when he suggested that we hold hands and pray with Mother. We circled her bed and held her hands in ours as we joined in the Lord's Prayer. She was not able to speak or even recognize us. But we knew that she was with us in spirit. Yes, she was very much present. She had a look of utter peace and contentment on her face as she left this earth with one big sigh. She taught everyone around her that dying can be normal, natural, peaceful and yes, even pleasant.

I have seen others die gently, but many, many more go through so much on the way out. Many remain in a vegetative state for months or years before they actually leave. It is sometimes hard to live in North America but it can be infinitely more difficult to die here. When the crisis occurs the family naturally turns to the doctor for advice about what to do. He may have absolutely no knowledge of the family's views on the issue. If he has not formulated his own philosophy about the meaning of life, he may be reluctant to discuss the issue at all. And once the life-saving machine starts rolling, there is little one can do to stop it. When the patient is all hooked up to the devices in a modern intensive care unit, it almost takes an act of Congress to turn off the equipment. I am reminded of an incident in our country where a frantic young father held off nurses at gun point. He wanted to remove his little son from the life support machines so the child could die in peace in his arms. That infant had been on machines for months. What was the hope of recovery? Why was the father forced to take such drastic measures in order to save his child from the system?

Death is not the end of anything. It is a transition to another plane of existence. All religious teachings agree on that. Why then do we refuse to accept it? We need to take a higher view. Our perspective must be changed. We must be clear about what we expect from the medical system. We need to assert our rights as consumers before the whole system is out of hand.

Not surprisingly, some alert and educated consumers

have begun to question this whole issue. Hence the emergence of groups of people who are lobbying for more freedom in directing their own lives right up to the end. Derek Humphrey founded the Hemlock Society which has forty chapters in the U.S. today. Members of this organization believe that if any person has been determined to be terminally ill and so certified by two medical doctors that the person has the right to medications which will end their suffering. Neither attempted suicide nor suicide are considered crimes in America but assisting someone to commit the act is. Therefore, even if a patient begs to be set free from his suffering, the law-abiding health care professional is forbidden to assist him.

Suicide is a highly emotional issue in our country and most people abhor the idea of it. But some have made a conscious decision to take that means if they feel forced to do so by advancing debility, pain and the expense of dying in America. They have free choice. It is their right to live and to die in any manner they choose.

The vast majority of people who *have* come to terms with their own mortality have discussed their ideas with their families and their physicians. Many have signed documents which are called "Living Wills". The main purpose of having these is to assure that their own preferences are respected if and when there is ever a question about whether or not to resuscitate them. It is important to address these issues far in advance of the time when decisions have to be made.

Most nurses I know would never opt for resuscitation and dramatic life-saving measures if they themselves were in a similar type of situation. A standard comment which I have heard is: "I think that I will have a tattoo put across my chest, DO NOT RESUSCITATE! If you guys ever put me through that I promise to come back and haunt you for the rest of your days!" If that is indeed the case, and you honestly do not want to have any heroics performed on you, then you'd better write it down. More important, you'd better let your doctor know how you feel.

How do we caregivers cope with the frustration of working within a system with views death as a failure? Well, we don't have a problem if we share that point of view. But most of the nurses I have known have a much more humane approach to the care of the critically ill. Since we are the ones who are at the bedside twenty-four hours a day, seven days a week, we have a good understanding of what that patient and family are going through. We are the ones who bring up the question of "Code status" because we are the ones who have to start giving the CPR* when Grandma breathes her last breath. We have to get all the emergency equipment and personnel into the room to resuscitate the dying patient even when it makes absolutely no sense to do so.

I believe that the most important role any health professional can play for her patient is that of advocate. So many people are unaware of how the system operates. It does not occur to them that even though Grandpa is terminally ill we have to intervene with life-saving measures when he stops breathing. It does not make sense to most people, so they don't think it is a possibility. They have no idea of just what a "code" entails. It is up to us to be open and willing to discuss all the aspects of patient care before the crisis occurs.

One really bright and beautiful spot in this whole gloomy picture is the Hospice movement. Hospice is a concept which was developed a number of years ago and which has brought to many people an opportunity to die with dignity. There is absolutely no reason why anyone needs to suffer unmanageable pain or misery at the time of death. In my

---

* CPR: cardiopulmonary resuscitation; a procedure designed to restore normal breathing after cardiac arrest that includes the clearance of air passages to the lungs, heart massage by the exertion of pressure on the chest, and the use of drugs.

practice, I have found that pain is the main fear for most. They can accept their dying if they are reassured that they do not have to die in agony. Hospice pioneered new methods of handling pain. Professionals who work in the Hospice area are dedicated to providing loving supportive care to patients right up to the end. Families are usually provided with support systems beyond the death itself and through the period of mourning and healing which must follow.

It is sometimes hard for families to get their loved ones into a Hospice program but it can be done. One family I worked with found that their doctor adamantly refused to admit the father to Hospice even though it was clearly what the patient wanted. Undaunted by the doctor's lack of cooperation, they sought and found a caring physician who was willing to take over the case. Their loved one was permitted a peaceful and comfortable exit because they demanded and got what he wanted at the time of his death.

Each caregiver must come to terms with the reality in which she works. She must make peace with the issues of death and dying. The only way that she can be empowered to do that is by nurturing her own spiritual Being. There are no mistakes. She is in that place at that time for a purpose, her own as well as her patient's. She needs to be as centered and serene about the meaning of life and death as she can possibly be. There is no other way for her to deal successfully with her work as a caregiver unless she develops a strong inner core of spirituality.

WORKBOOK EXERCISE

End of Chapter Fourteen.

Answer the following questions "Yes" or "No."

1. I am comfortable in the presence of a dying patient:

2. I realize that death is an important part of life:

3. I have read and enjoyed the work of Elisabeth Kubler-Ross:

4. I have a deep spiritual connection:

5. I never have any difficulty bringing up the subject of Code Status with my patients/clients:

6. I spend as much time with my dying patients/clients as I do with the rest of my patients/clients:

7. I have experienced the death of someone close to me:

8. I have no fear of my own death:

9. I have questioned the health care value system in our society:

10. I have a problem participating on the Code team when we have to resuscitate the frail elderly or severely handicapped patient who has expressed a desire to die:

If you have answered "No" to three or more of the above questions you may wish to explore the issue of death and dying further.

1. Consider reading one or more of the books at the end of this chapter.

2. Discuss your discomfort and/or fears with a person you respect either in the health care field or the ministry.

3. Go within, in meditation and ask your Higher Self to assist you with getting into a peaceful mindframe about death and dying.

FURTHER READING

Butterworth, Eric. *Discover the Power Within You.* (Harper & Row, 1989). An inspiring work on spirituality which includes a section on the theory of reincarnation.

A Course in Miracles. (Foundation for Inner Peace, 1975).

Humphry, Derek. *Final Exit: The Practicalities of Self-Deliverance and Assisted Suicide for the Dying* (Hemlock Society, 1991). Discusses terminal illness and rational suicide, and offers guidance to those supporting this option.

Kubler-Ross, Elisabeth. *Death: The Final Stage of Growth* (Prentice-Hall, 1975). Kubler-Ross, Elisabeth. *On Death and Dying* (Macmillan, 1972). The writings of Elisabeth Kubler-Ross explain the dying process and show that there is nothing to fear from the experience.

Chapter 15: The Long Voyage Home

The Search for God

If you cannot hear the Voice of God, it is because you do not choose to listen.

– A Course in Miracles

Be strong and of good courage; be not frightened neither be dismayed; for the Lord your God is with you wherever you go.

– Joshua 1: 9

There are many, many methods of getting in touch with the God within. Humans have discovered that in a great variety of ways down through the ages. We all have a Divine guidance system, of that there is no doubt. For some of us the voice is nearly obscured by our emotions and materialism. But it is still there. It is simply waiting to be nurtured into full flowering force in our lives.

We caregivers must learn to follow the inner Direction which leads to serenity in a seemingly chaotic world if we are going to be able to function well in our present health-care system. I believe that the frustration and despair which lead to burn-out could be averted altogether if we learned how to nurture and develop our inner Being and strength.

One of the very best ways to begin the search for inner peace is through regular physical exercise. This may sound odd, but it really is true. I found that when I ran for three miles without stopping, my body automatically put me into a different state of mind. I found it easier to access my deep inner thoughts, beliefs, fears, and hopes while I was working out. I am not at all sure why this is so, but I have read many other accounts of runners who say that this is true. It seems so natural to think about spiritual ideas and values when we running or walking. Communication with our Higher Power comes easily when we are surrounded by His incredible handiwork

Quite by accident, I discovered what many people had learned before me. When we take steps to enhance one area of our lives, we automatically improve function in the other two. Therefore, I found that as I became more physically fit, both my spiritual and emotional fitness improved as well. Never will I voluntarily abandon my exercise program. I may need to modify it somewhat over time, but I cannot give it up. It makes me feel tuned into the universe and God's love for me.

One of the basic principles of holistic health is that we cannot separate our physical body from out emotional, mental and spiritual states of being.

– Shakti Gawain

What Shakti Gawain says is so true and yet so misunderstood by so many. I have heard caregivers complain about fatigue and depression for years. When I suggest that they try physical exercise to combat their feeling low, they look at me in disbelief. "I work so hard now and yet you say that I should go out and walk when I get home!" But they try it and are amazed to discover a sense of well being which had previously eluded them. They begin to glow and smile as they go about the same hard work they were doing before. They report having found a sense of inner peace and contentment which they thought they had lost forever. Exercise makes all the difference in my life. Time and again I have seen it work just as well for others.

Another method which helped me to get in touch with my Higher Self was to begin journaling regularly. It began when

I was in turmoil of the ending of my marriage. I was thinking about starting over in a new place, far away from my home. Each night I wrote about my feelings, explored my options, and expressed my needs. I found my self getting closer and closer to the inner Being. That was not my goal when I began, but what a wonderful benefit it turned out to be.

Since that time I have journaled regularly. When I look back on what I felt and revealed to myself along the way, I can see so clearly how far I've come on the path. I have a long way to go, and I choose to continue learning and growing forever. Working away at the problems is sort of like peeling away the layers of an onion: sometimes it makes us cry. Expressing everything honestly clarifies our thoughts. When I have felt particularly perplexed about a problem I have followed the advice of Donna McClure who recommends "journaling letters to God."

Donna is a licensed Unity Teacher who expresses her God-self exquisitely as she works. She learned to write a letter to God at bedtime, pouring out her heart and soul in an honest revelation of what she felt and needed during a time of real challenge. The next morning without reading what she had written the night before, she wrote a letter to Donna from God. The message came from her heart without being filtered first through her intellect. The results were quite marvelous. Her God within was able to advise her easily and clearly on all of her questions. And, her God-self revealed tremendous love and support for her. Donna recommends this type of journaling for anyone who is in need of clarification and centering. Of course that fits all of us some of the time. I have tried it and been astonished at how very well it works. I endorse the idea heartily. Try it for a week and you will be amazed at how it helps you to get a handle on what is really happening and what steps you can take to overcome your problems. It is potentially a life-changing exercise and well worth the effort.

Ever since humans appeared on earth, we knew that there was a Force which was in charge. To my knowledge there is no tribe or group which does not worship some concept of God. It is the powerful drive toward a connection with God which brings us all to our knees in adoration and supplication. Prayer works. Obviously it does, or we would have stopped doing it eons ago!

When I was a child I was taught to pray using rote formulas or prayer books. Once in a while I use this method as a sort of prayer mantra or blessing. More often though I just close my eyes and speak to God in my own words. I have found great comfort in prayer as I know others do. We may all do it differently but the important thing is doing it. The simplest and most important prayer is "Thank you God!"

One thing we must understand is that God is not some nebulous entity floating "Out There" somewhere. God is within each and every one of us.

God is everything and everywhere. God is infinite Love and Understanding. God is the only Force active in the universe and we are all a part of Him and a part of His plan. But we have got to get in touch with Him in order to express Him freely in our lives. It is up to us; He never moves away from us. It is we who move away from Him. Daily prayer is important for good spiritual health.

Talking to God is a firm cornerstone upon which to build a strong spiritual connection. Listening to God, through meditation is another powerful way to get in touch with the Divine Force within us. It is not an easy thing for Western man to quiet the hustle and bustle of a busy world in order to listen to the Inner Voice, but as many will agree, it can be done. Meditation has been promoted as a powerful spiritual tool by Eastern religious teachers for many generations. There is nothing difficult about doing it. One simply must find a quiet spot, get into a comfortable sitting position, relax all parts of the body and pay attention to the rhythms of

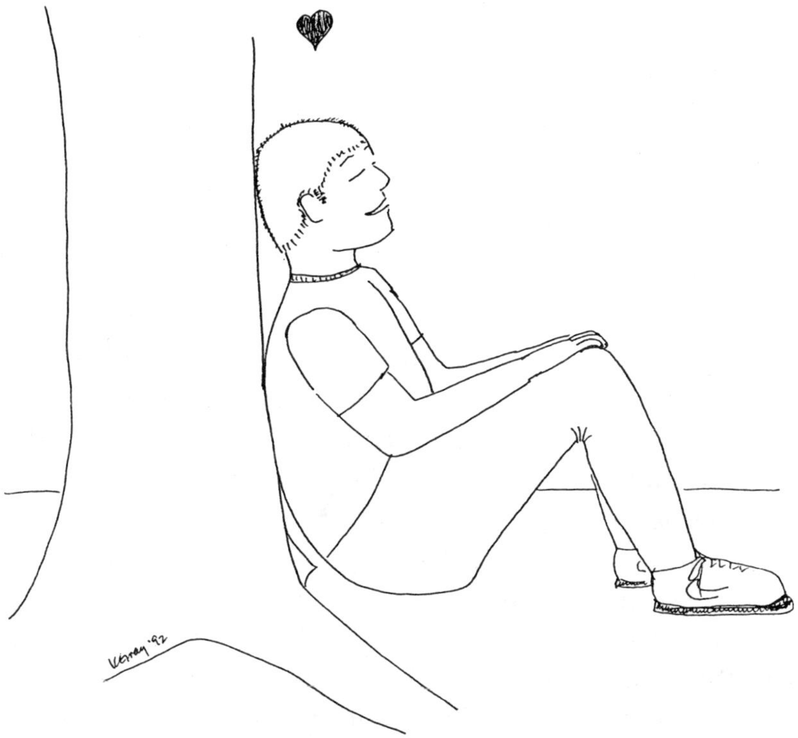

breathing. Clearing the mind of all thoughts is the goal. As thoughts appear in the consciousness, they need to be dismissed. Concentrate on the breathing. Pay attention to whatever visions or messages arrive. If nothing meaningful comes, that is fine. It is rather like allowing muddy water to settle. When the water is allowed to get very still, it invariably will clarify. Once we are clear, we can hear the Voice.

Try meditating for short periods at first. Ten minutes is fine. As it becomes easier to get peaceful and centered, we can meditate for longer and longer periods. One Buddhist man I know meditates easily for an hour or more every day. He says he has no idea of the passage of time. Meditation is something I can do anywhere or anytime. Where I have enjoyed it the most is near the ocean where I could get a sense of God's presence and power from the crashing waves. There I could sit for long periods of time. The soft, warm wind on my face felt like a gentle caress of a loving God. Today I meditate in my home, in a quiet spot and that works just as well.

Joseph Campbell said that all of life is meditation. That is certainly true, so long as we keep the thought of God uppermost in our minds as we go through the day. As we feel that Power within us, we are free to let go of the fears that bind us to our self-defeating behaviors and thoughts.

Our thoughts have far more energy than we realize. They are real entities and whatever we focus on gets bigger and more powerful with each moment. That is why it is critical for us to think and speak positive, uplifting ideas rather than negative, heavy ones. When a negative thought comes into the mind, we release it immediately and reframe it in a positive, affirming way.

Affirmations are another powerful tool for getting in touch with our inner Strength. We can use them in many different ways. What they do, of course, is reprogram our subconscious mind in a much more positive direction. In order to increase our personal power it helps us to use affirmations on a regular basis. Here are some which have been very useful to me:

I AM A BELOVED CHILD OF GOD.

I AM ENTITLED TO ALL ABUNDANCE IN LOVE, HEALTH, PEACE AND PROSPERITY.

I HAVE EVERYTHING I NEED.

I HAVE ALL WISDOM AND UNDERSTANDING WITHIN ME.

I EXPRESS ONLY LOVE AND TRUTH

I AM ONE WITH MOTHER EARTH AND ALL HER INHABITANTS

I TRUST THE GOD WITHIN ME TO LEAD ME WHEREVER I NEED TO GO.

WITH THE HELP OF GOD I NOW MANIFEST THE PERFECT PLAN FOR MY LIFE.

PERFECT PEACE IS MINE

I AM HEALTHY, WHOLE AND COMPLETE.

GOD LOVES ME.

Make up your own affirmations. The important thing is that they keep you in touch with a Power greater than your ego-self. We are so much more than just flesh and blood. We may look like solid matter, dense human form, but in essence we are beings of Light who have chosen to manifest in this form in order to learn our lessons here on the earth.

Though we may look different from one another, in our essence we are all one. That can be a frightening thought when we look at people who are acting out in negative ways, but it is true. Those who are difficult to like are manifesting different aspects of our personalities. We find ourselves reacting to them only because we see our own negative qualities in them, whether or not we realize that. They are our teachers. We must thank them for helping us learn more about ourselves. When we accept them, even on an inner level, thanking them for what they are teaching us, we release them from affecting us anymore.

Only when you turn within and feel God can you begin to see God in others.

– Nana Veary

We can express our God-selves more clearly and joyfully in our work, our personal lives and in our play. All we need to do is nurture that very special part of us which lifts up from the mundane and into the light.

There is....one God and Father for us all, who is above all and through all and IN all.

– Ephesians 4:6

WORKBOOK EXERCISE

End of Chapter Fifteen

Answer the following questions with "Yes" or "No"

1. I can easily see the presence of God in everyone:

2. I get a sense of peace and comfort from prayer:

3. Doing affirmations helps me to develop my spiritual connection:

4. Journaling is a useful tool for me to get in touch with my inner self:

5. I journal on a daily basis:

6. I meditate regularly:

7. I notice a sense of spiritual connection when I am running, walking, cycling, or just active outdoors:

8. I wish I could spend more time in prayer and meditation:

9. I feel the presence of God within me:

10. I am very happy with my religious affiliation:

If you have answered "No" to three or more of the above questions you may want to do one or more of the following exercises:

1. Begin journaling on a daily basis. Try Donna's method of pouring out your heart to God at night and then responding with a letter to yourself from God in the morning.

2. Set aside thirty minutes a day for prayer and meditation with some spiritual reading.

3. Notice the good in other people. Pay attention to the expressions of kindness and caring for others. See the God in them.

4. Notice the good in yourself. Pay attention to the many ways you express love and caring in your daily work and in your personal life. See the God within you.

If you commit to the above exercises you will see an amazing difference in the quality of your life by the end of a week. Keep it up. Your life will improve beyond all expectations.

FURTHER READING

Fields, Rick, and Taylor, Peggy. *Chop Wood, Carry Water: A Guide to Finding Spiritual Fulfillment in Everyday Life.* (St. Martin's, 1984).

Fox, Emmet. *Diagrams for Living: The Bible Unveiled.* (Harper & Row, 1968). A tool for rediscovering the wisdom in the Bible.

Fox, Emmet. *Find and Use Your Inner Power.* (Harper & Row, 1941). Based on the belief that the will of God for man/woman is freedom, health and harmony, and that these things can be attained by learning the laws of life and applying them.

Goldsmith, Joel. *God, the Substance of All Form.* (Citadel Press, 1962). A manual for applying universal spiritual truth for health, healing and daily life.

Harp, David. *The Three-Minute Meditator.* (New Harbinger, 1990). A tool for beginners in meditation.

Kushner, Harold. *Who Needs God?* (Summit Books, 1989). Explains the positive benefits of having a relationship with God. The author's other writings include *When Bad Things Happen to Good People*.

LeShan, Lawrence. *How to Meditate: A Guide to Self-Discovery*. (Bantam, 1986). Simply written introductory text on the philosophy and practice of meditation.

Ram Dass. *Journey of Awakening: A Meditator's Guidebook*. (Bantam, 1978). An introduction to meditation by the author of *Be Here Now*.

Chapter 16: Putting it all Together

Review and Summary

The work-place allows you to challenge illusions, come face to face with a great many fears and to find the gifts and talents you have.

– Emmanuel

Finally you understand that the real motorcycle you're working on is yourself.

– Robert Pirsig

Who cares for the caregiver? That job rests with the caregiver herself. She must not abdicate responsibility for her own nurturing to anyone else. She must not assume that others will know how to help her. She must learn to speak her truth honestly and courageously. There is no need to run away from professions which offer many opportunities for service, happiness and personal growth.

Each one of us must view ourselves as a pitcher of cool, clear water. In order to pour out and serve others, we must keep the pitcher full. We cannot give when there is nothing in the container. If we care so little about ourselves that we become exhausted and depleted, how can we help others?

Our primary responsibility is first to love ourselves. That means we must identify our needs and speak our truth. We must stand up for our rights. Shall we give over our own nurturing to the institution? Can we expect a huge medical center or even a small agency to understand what we as individuals need unless we tell them?

We must decide what it is we need and want in the workplace and then create that reality for ourselves. No more complaining and groaning without taking action. Look at the messages you give your employer. Are you willing to feel overburdened, abused, harassed? Do not wait until you can't take it anymore. Speak up. Band together. Take care of yourselves.

Go within. Examine your goals, your dreams. Decide how you want to manage your life. Speak your truth. Find the best way to express your love and talents. There are many, many different options available. Find the one which suits you. Don't abandon your profession because you lack the courage to express your needs. No one else will know what you want unless you tell them.

Take care of yourself. Let go of your addictions. Cope with life openly and honestly. You are a beloved child of God. You deserve to be happy. Get into good physical condition. You will be surprised how much more enjoyable and tolerable your life will be when you are in a state of high-level wellness. Stress is far more manageable when you are healthy.

Get enough rest. No more of this super-woman behavior. You don't have to carry the weight of the world on your shoulders. Tell people how they can help you. Don't expect them to guess. Enlist the support of colleagues, spouse, family and children. Open your mouth and speak your truth.

Do things you really love doing. Don't allow yourself to be propelled by guilt and fear. Be your own judge and be your own advocate. Who cares what the rest of the world thinks? It is none of your business what they think about you. It is your life. If you don't live it the way you want to, you have only yourself to blame.

Don't get trapped in codependent relationships which deplete you of all of your energy. You deserve to have a partner who is loving, supportive, nurturing and caring. If you find yourself doing all the giving in the relationship, there is something wrong. You can't make someone love you. Someone either loves you or does not. Hanging around with

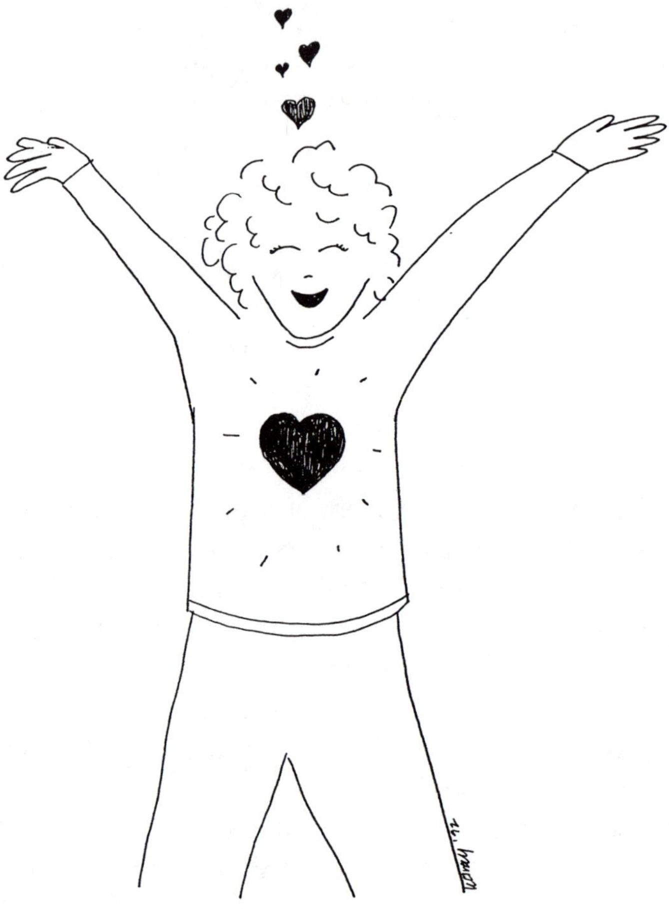

people who are abusive and uncaring is destructive and unhealthy. There are so many wonderful people out there.

Take responsibility for your own happiness. Don't expect someone else to do it for you. You are in charge of your own growth in this world. It is your journey; you are not responsible for anyone else's path. Live your life fully, honestly, courageously. Face your fears. Avoiding the things you fear will not help you to evolve. The only way to grow is to move right into your fear, experience it and master it. Or to paraphrase a recent book on the subject, feel the fear and get on with it anyway. After all, you came here to learn and grow.

Create beauty and wellness in all areas of your life. Make sure that you express the unique being that is you. You don't have to believe everything that you see in women's magazines, or men's magazines, for that matter! Love the being that you are. You created that body, that face. It is perfect. You are beautiful and special just the way you are.

Create a lovely, peaceful environment in which to live. It does not have to be expensive . You do not have to spend great piles of money. You will feel so much better if you have a place which feels good to you, which expresses who you are. Decorate your place with the colors which make you feel good, with pictures which cause you to relax and be peaceful. Put up photos of the people and places that you love. Play music which brings joy and serenity to your being.

Be in charge of your life. Learn to say "No" and mean it. It will feel strange at first, but each time you do it, it will become easier. Remember that your first allegiance must be to yourself. You will do no one else any good if you forget that and burn out. If you don't like the job you have and cannot make changes there which will make it more pleasant, find a different job. Take the chance.

Creating security in this world is an illusion. The more we grasp at it, the more it eludes us. If we fear making changes we lock ourselves in a corner and limit our experience. Trust your Higher Power to guide and take care of you. The more you nurture your spiritual self, the stronger it will get and the more you will understand that there is absolutely nothing to fear.

Promote emotional wellness by developing your serenity. Inner peace will be yours when you let go of your destructive habits and love your body, mind and spirit. Learn to meditate and to pray. Learn to enjoy solitude, be outdoors in nature, be alone and not lonely. Be open to your intuition, your inner Guide. Love yourself with all your heart. Only when you have come to that unconditional self-acceptance, will you be able to accept others as they are.

Take advantage of all the wonderful books which have been written by gifted teachers (don't forget to try the library first!). Read and learn. Join a support group in order to have the help you need so you can overcome your difficulties. Learn how to play, to enjoy your life. It is a great adventure. There are no mistakes. Some paths are more difficult than others, but all the lessons are for our highest good. Remain in the present and live one day at a time.

You came into this life with a mission to accomplish; it is no accident that you are a caregiver. You have been guided to serve others in a very special way. Take care of the caregiver so that she can continue to express her unique gifts to all of mankind. Love her, support her, protect her. She is a very special being, much cherished by the Almighty and by her fellow humans on this journey.

Merle Shain sums it up very well with the following thought:

There are really only two ways to approach life - as a victim or a gallant fighter - and you must decide if you want to act or react, deal your own cards or play with a stacked deck. And if you don't decide which way to play with life, it always plays with you.

Appendix

Support Organizations:

Alcoholics Anonymous. Box 459 Grand Central Station New York NY 10163

Alanon Family Groups Headquarters. P.O. Box 862 Midtown Station NewYork NY 10018-0862 (212) 302-7240.

Alateen. P.O. Box 862 Midtown Station New York NY 10018-0862

Co-dependents Anonymous. P.O. Box 33577 Phoenix AZ 85067-3577 (602) 277-7991.

Codependents Anonymous for Health Professionals. P.O. Box 18191 Mesa AZ 85212 (602) 971-3284

Co-Sex Addicts Anonymous. P.O. Box 1453 Minneapolis MN 55414

Debtors Anonymous. P.O. Box 20322 New York NY 10025-999 (212) 642-8220.

Emotional Health Anonymous. 2420 San Gabriel Blvd. Rosemead CA 91770 (818) 573-5482.

Emotions Anonymous. P.O. Box 4245 St. Paul MN 55104 (612) 647-9712

International Nurses Anonymous. (415) 386-3014

Narcotics Anonymous. P.O. Box 9999 Van Nuys CA 91409 (818) 780-3951

National Self-Help Clearinghouse. 25 W. 43rd St. Room 620 New York NY 10036 (212) 642-2944

Overachievers Anonymous. 1777 Union St. San Francisco CA 94123 (415) 928-3600.

Overeaters Anonymous. P.O. Box 92870 Los Angeles CA 90009 (213) 542-8363.

Sex Addicts Anonymous. P.O.Box 3038 Minneapolis MN 55403 (612) 339-0127.

Sex and Love Addicts Anonymous P.O. Box 119 New Town Branch Boston MA 02258 (617) 332-1845.

Smokers Anonymous. 2118 Greenwich St. San Francisco CA 94128 (415) 922-8575.

Workaholics Anonymous. 75 Grasslands Rd. Valhalla NY 1059

Appendix

Associations:

International Medical & Dental Hypnotherapy Association. 4110 Edgeland Suite 800 Royal Oak MI 48073

National Clearinghouse for Alcohol Information. P.O. Box 2345 Rockville MD 20852 (301) 468-2600

National Council on Alcoholism and Drug Dependence. 12 W. 21st. St. Seventh Floor New York NY 10010 (212) 206-6770

National Council on Compulsive Gambling. 445 W. 59th St. New York NY (212) 765-3833

Index

Index

Index

Index

Index

Index

Index

Index

About the Author

Roberta Jarrett was born in Canada and received her diploma in nursing from the St. Boniface Hospital School of Nursing in Manitoba. She earned a certificate for teaching and supervision in schools of nursing from the University of Manitoba. She later received her BSN from Moorhead State University. She also holds a diploma in Hypnotherapy from the Wesland Institute. She has been a practicing clinical nurse for more than three decades, working in areas of staff nursing, teaching, and nursing management. Her recent experience includes positions at the Queen's Medical Center and the Rehabilitation Hospital of the Pacific in Honolulu.

Ms. Jarrett devotes her time to writing, speaking and leading workshops on the subject of high level wellness, traveling regularly to major cities in the U.S. and Canada. Her writings include articles for *Nursing Success Today* and *Compendium*. **Caring for the Caregiver** is her first book. A second book, **Kalaupapa Diary**, which chronicles her experience at the Hansen's Disease Settlement in Kalaupapa, Hawaii, will be published in the Spring of 1993. She currently lives with her husband Bryan in Beaverton, Oregon.

About the Illustrator

Katherine Gray was born in North Dakota and graduated with a Bachelor's degree from the University of North Dakota. She currently works as a freelance artist and writer in San Diego.

Order Form

Please send ________ copies of **Caring for the Caregiver.**

Price: US$12.95; CAN$14.95
Add $2.00 per copy postage & handling.
[Bank check, money order or personal check accepted. No cash or COD, please].
Group and bulk rates also available.

For VISA or MasterCard complete below: ______________________

Visa #: ______________________ Expires: ______________

MC #: ______________________ Expires: ______________

Cardholder's Signature: ______________________________

Name: ____

Address: ____

City: ________________ State: ________ Zip Code: ____________

Information on workshops, classes, retreats, and speaking engagements available. Write or call:

PACIFIC EDITIONS
11838 S.W. WINDMILL DR.
BEAVERTON, OR 97005
TEL : (503) 526-9720

Contact Person: Bryan Stoneburner